Supervision and Support in Primary Care

Edited by

Jonathan Burton

Associate Dean
Department of Postgraduate GP Education
London Deanery

and

John Launer

Senior Lecturer in General Practice and Primary Care
Tavistock Clinic

Radcliffe Medical Press

Radcliffe Medical Press Ltd
18 Marcham Road
Abingdon
Oxon OX14 1AA
United Kingdom

www.radcliffe-oxford.com
The Radcliffe Medical Press electronic catalogue and online ordering facility.
Direct sales to anywhere in the world.

British Library Cataloguing in Publication Data

A catalogue record for this book is available from the British Library.

ISBN 1 85775 951 6

Typeset by Aarontype Ltd, Easton, Bristol
Printed and bound by TJ International Ltd, Padstow, Cornwall

Contents

Preface

The book has arisen out of a friendship and a working partnership. We are both general practitioners (GPs) who have been in practice for more than 20 years, although in very different localities. We both enjoy our work greatly, and we retain our enthusiasm for primary care as a place where important and effective human encounters can take place. We also regard primary care as an unusually complex and challenging setting for professionals, where most perform a remarkable job under significant pressure – nearly always with very limited resources for clinical supervision and support. We hope that this book will help to make the case for greatly expanding those resources. We share a belief that such an expansion could encourage recruitment, enhance job satisfaction, maintain and elevate professional standards, and – perhaps most crucially – protect against stress and burn out in the primary care professions.

Our professional paths crossed originally because of a shared interest in post-graduate education for primary care. We were each engaged in developing roles as primary care educators: one as an associate dean for the London region, now mainly responsible for developing educational research; and the other as a senior lecturer at the Tavistock Clinic. For several years now, we have joined together in organising an annual conference at the Tavistock Clinic on the topic of 'Working models of supervision and support in primary care', supported by the North London Education and Training Consortium. These conferences have evolved over the years from a mainly auditorium-based exposition on the various models of supervision and support available in primary care, to a far more experiential approach in which participants elected to join workshops to try out a variety of different approaches. We have learnt a great deal from these conferences, and in particular from the formal evaluation of the 2001 event (Souster 2001). The views of participants – a mixed group of clinicians, educators, managers and mental health professionals – have contributed a great deal to our thinking about this book. Almost all the authors in this book have contributed to these conferences as presenters or workshop leaders.

As well as our involvement in the Tavistock conferences, we have also both been members of an informal forum that was set up in 1995, called the Innovations in Education Research Group (IERG). Members of this group are mostly educators and facilitators themselves (as well as being doctors, nurses and researchers by core profession). The purpose of the group has been to provide a forum not only for discussing different approaches to educational research but also for providing mutual support for its members. The group's work has involved research into the culture of primary care, new approaches to learning, such as self-directed learning groups and multiprofessional, problem-based learning, and into how mature practitioners can best learn about the consultation. These studies have been well disposed to the difficulties of primary care. Much of the thinking in this book is informed by the work of IERG, and altogether seven chapter authors in this book are or have been members of that group, including Linden West who led it for a number of years.

Our interest as educators has never been exclusively with clinical supervision of the kinds described in this book. It has been with the whole spectrum of activities that can help people working in primary care with their professional and personal development. The spectrum extends from formal courses aimed at teaching specific skills, to sudden, unexpected interactions with colleagues and patients that may lead to new enlightenment or sustained growth. However, two factors in particular have led us to produce a book with the specific focus of clinical supervision and support.

The first of these has been our contact with professions outside primary care, particular in the mental health field and social work, where clinical supervision is well established and is seen as a prerequisite for ethical and competent practice. These professions bring wholly different perspectives to their daily work, and yet their work is sometimes very similar to the work of GPs and primary care nurses. For this reason, we dedicate considerable space on this book to describing the concept of supervision in mental health practice. We do not take an idealised view of supervision in these professions, nor do we assume that everything that applies there can and should be transferred to primary care. We recognise that, for most primary care practitioners, imitating this type of supervision may be impracticable and possibly inappropriate. However, one of our aims in editing this book has been to give readers an opportunity to consider what might be learnt from these professions, especially from how they support their members in dealing with the challenges of their everyday work.

The other factor that has influenced us is the accelerating change in the UK in the last few years towards a culture of public accountability in the primary care professions. We take an educational rather than a service management view and are therefore keen to differentiate between clinical supervision and support, on the one hand, and monitoring processes such as appraisal and revalidation, on the other. Nevertheless, people in primary care now work within a professional and social context where legitimate concerns about professional standards of practice cannot be ignored. Our own view is that clinical supervision and support is potentially more effective than external assessment in raising and maintaining professional standards, and in protecting the public. We believe it is important to research, develop and promote voluntary methods of clinical supervision and support forms of activity that are superior in many ways to forms of policing. This is a theme that runs, implicitly and explicitly, through the whole book.

Our own views have evolved considerably in the course of compiling this book. When we started the project, we differed considerably in our understanding of what supervision meant. One of us (JB), working entirely within primary care and primary care education, understood it to mean a very wide range of activities, including many of the conversations that take place every day in surgeries and clinics. The other (JL), trained as a therapist as well as a GP, took a more rigorous and formal view of what did and did not qualify as supervision. Through working together, we have both moved towards the middle ground in our thinking. Each of us has come to recognise that clinical supervision needs to be approached with both an openness to innovation and variety, and also with some clear sense of boundaries. Some echoes of our original differences may possibly still resonate in these pages and we make no apology for this. Like us, readers will each need to explore and define their own positions in relation to the need for supervision in primary care, and the forms it should take. We see this book as an attempt to promote debate rather than to propose dogma.

In many hours of discussion with each other and with the chapter authors, we have come to realise that there exists within primary care a whole range of activities that, to differing degrees, is providing supervision and support. Many of these activities have not been recognised as having this purpose, as they have usually been convened in the first place for the purposes of learning. Others are easily recognisable as supervision or support. In the book, we have tried to cover a spectrum of activity. For example, we look at clinical supervision in nursing, which often follows a fairly rigorous approach. We also look at some of the more haphazard approaches that have grown up in primary care settings over the last few years. There are many stages in between. Individuals or supervision groups may well move in and out of different types of experience, and some chapters in the book reflect this fact too.

The different authors in this book do not use the term 'supervision' in identical ways, and we have not tried to harmonise their contributions in a vain attempt to present 'consensus' around definitions or principles. A constant theme of this book is that supervision cannot be seen as one single concrete method or approach that is entirely separate and distinguishable from everything else. Indeed, a number of authors in this book avoid the term 'supervision' almost entirely, whereas others stress that supervision is simply one aspect of what they do, or one among several ways of understanding their approach. Some of the authors place supervision alongside the facilitation of learning of knowledge, skills and attitudes. Others see it more as a different entity. Some of the chapters describe clearly defined theoretical ideas, structures or methodologies; others are more concerned with overall attitudes. Similarly, some of the chapters are personal and passionate accounts, written in the first person, whereas others present more formal or official arguments. We value the diversity of the approaches to clinical supervision represented here, both from within and outside primary care. We believe that many different descriptions of clinical supervision are better than one and we think it is important not to promote any one of them as the only 'right' way. We are happy to offer readers a range of different ideas and methods, and to leave them to form their own views about each of them. What we are concerned to promote is a culture of regular, sustained and reflective learning in relation to the everyday work in primary care – by whatever means this happens.

Whilst the main purpose or end-point of supervision is the development of professional competence, we also want to emphasise the supportive nature of any relationship that enables practitioners to function well generally and to avoid stress and burn out. So we have included chapters on forms of professional interaction that are based more exclusively on the concept of nurturing or support, such as mentorship, co-tutoring, and self-directed learning groups. We recognise that there is a seamless connection between support, supervision, reflective practice and having a 'learning workplace'. We do not want to set up an over-rigid distinction between these and 'proper' supervision.

In the pages that follow, therefore, we introduce many different views of what clinical supervision entails, and a number of separate specific models involving an aspect of supervision or support. We invite readers to enter into dialogue with each of the authors, and to consider what they might or might not want to incorporate into their own thinking or practice. In particular, we would like to ask people to imagine ways in which these various approaches to supervision, from within the primary care professions or outside them, might be adapted to normal life in the surgery, health centre or community clinic – and how they might be turned into core activities rather than haphazard ones. One of our preoccupations in the book is with how primary care might develop its own 'native' methods of supervision and support, taking on some of the relevant practices of different professions, but developing others for itself. We also want to invite readers to think about the questions: 'What is the place of formal structures and methodologies in clinical supervision? Is the lack of these in primary care a strength, a weakness, or a bit of both?'

Through years of contact with very many other colleagues, in both clinical and educational settings, we have learnt of the various ways that people in primary care develop as practitioners and as people. We edit this book in that knowledge, and in the personal knowledge of what has helped us change from what we were to what we are as practitioners now – however imperfect that may be. We know that the contributions in this book are by no means exhaustive. They are reports on types of supervision and support with which we have had direct contact. We are aware of others that are not covered in these pages, but which many readers will be aware of. Nevertheless, we hope that the range of activities covered here, and the way they are described, will help to promote a fertile and continuing discussion about the need for clinical supervision and support in primary care, and about the various forms that this might take.

The shape of the book

The book is in four parts.

Part I is called 'Claiming the territory'. It consists of three introductory chapters by the editors, setting out the area of the book, looking at the nature and purpose of clinical supervision, and discussing how to raise its profile in primary care.

Part II offers two differing perspectives from the world of mental health. The first is a view from two psychotherapists, Helen West and Linden West, based on their experiences in a wide range of settings, including primary care. This is followed by an essay by Andrew Cooper, dean of postgraduate studies at the Tavistock Clinic, looking specifically at how to make supervision a supportive activity rather than a persecutory one.

Part III is the longest part of the book. It presents five different practical approaches, all written by primary care clinicians with extensive experience of developing methods of supervision and support for their colleagues working at the 'coal face'. It covers clinical supervision for practice nurses, Balint groups, narrative approaches, mentoring and co-tutoring, and self-directed learning groups.

Part IV looks at opportunities for introducing clinical supervision into GP postgraduate training. There is a chapter by Tareq Abouharb and Neil Jackson from the London GP deanery, addressing the political and administrative issues that surround the introduction of higher professional education for young GPs. The book ends with an essay by John Launer looking at how clinical supervision can be integrated into GP vocational training.

Jonathan Burton
John Launer
January 2003

Reference

Souster V (2001) *An Evaluation of the 'Working Models of Support and Supervision' Conference.* (www.londondeanery.ac.uk/gp/home.htm)

About the authors

The editors

Jonathan Burton
Associate Dean
Department of Postgraduate GP Education
London Deanery
General Practitioner

John Launer
Senior Clinical Lecturer and Honorary Consultant in General Practice
and Primary Care
Child and Family Department
Tavistock Clinic
General Practitioner

The contributors

Tareq Abouharb
Associate Dean for New GPs
Department of GP Education and Training
London Deanery
General Practitioner

Andrew Cooper
Professor of Social Work
Tavistock Clinic and University of East London
Dean of Postgraduate Studies
Tavistock and Portman NHS Trust

Sylvia Debreczeny
Associate Dean (CPD)
Department of GP Education and Training
London Deanery

Steve Hiew
Associate Dean of Postgraduate GP Education
London Deanery
General Practitioner

Neil Jackson
Dean of Postgraduate GP Education
London Deanery

Paul Paxton
Facilitator of East Anglian Co-Tutoring Scheme
General Practitioner

Paul Sackin
Course Organiser for Vocational Training Scheme
Co-Tutoring Facilitator
General Practitioner

John Salinsky
Course Organiser for Whittington Hospital GP Vocational Training Scheme
General Secretary, International Balint Federation
General Practitioner

Nalliah Sivananthan
Educational Lead for PCT
Honorary Primary Care Tutor
General Practitioner

Helen West
Senior Lecturer in Education
Canterbury Christ Church, University College

Linden West
Principal Lecturer in Education
Canterbury Christ Church, University College

Acknowledgements

The idea for the book arose from a series of one-day conferences at the Tavistock Clinic, which we jointly organised. We would like to thank those who supported these conferences, especially Andrew Harris and Neil Jackson (representing the North London Consortium and the London Deanery, respectively) who saw the benefits of spreading the word about supervision in primary care. We would also like to thank our colleagues in the Innovations in Education Research Group (IERG). Some of the earlier work of Madeleine Reiss, Kathryn Burton, Linden West, Steve Hiew, Nalliah Sivananthan and Penny Morris (all members of or occasional attenders at the group) contributed greatly to our understanding of the need for supervision and support in primary care. The evaluation of the 2001 Tavistock Conference by Vicky Souster was presented in the group and discussed, and again helped us in the development of our thinking. We would like to thank all the chapter authors for their work and for their forbearance with us when we have asked them to consider changes.

We would like to acknowledge the untiring support of our personal assistants at the London Deanery (Pam Roue) and the Tavistock Clinic (Lucy Ettinger). We thank them for their help. Gillian Nineham has been a fantastically encouraging editor and has been generous in giving her time to this project. This has included joining us for meetings in London. This leads us to another acknowledgement – to The Kings Head in Winchmore Hill, London, where we have met from time to time over a period of a year. These meetings have represented a long and continuing debate about supervision and support in primary care, and an exploration of issues which are in some instances new and in other instances much better-understood by others.

Lastly, we thank our wives, Kathryn Burton and Lee Wax, for reading and commentating on our own writings for the book, for discussing various ideas with us, and for allowing us to work undisturbed for long periods of time.

Claiming the territory

CHAPTER 1

Primary care and the need for clinical supervision and support

Jonathan Burton and John Launer

In this book, we want to claim a territory for clinical supervision and support in primary care, a different territory from that occupied by much training and education, and by most performance appraisal. It is a territory that can be summed up by the phrase: 'professional enhancement'.

What is supervision?

Supervision is a particular kind of professional conversation. It is not the kind of conversation that involves giving people advice, assessing them or solving their problems for them. It is the kind that happens when you provide space, time and professional support for colleagues so that they can reflect on their encounters with patients or with colleagues. This sense of the word is recognised widely within many professions, including counselling, clinical psychology and social work. It is now starting to become familiar in primary care, where it is taking over from the more traditional understanding of the word as something managerial or hierarchical. Supervision in this sense is about looking after people rather than looking over their shoulders. In this book, we hope to promote the use of the word in this way. Most of all we hope to promote the activity it describes.

Supervision can happen in all sorts of ways. It can take place between two colleagues or in groups. The people involved may be equals or in a hierarchical relationship with each other. They might be from the same profession or different ones. Supervision can also happen in all kinds of settings: in managed environments, like nursing departments in trusts, or in decentralised settings, such as general practices. It can occur in sessions that are formally described as supervision, but it can also arise during other kinds of activities that go under different names. Sometimes it occurs in a training context: so-called 'educational supervision'. Whatever form supervision takes, the common denominator is that it offers an opportunity for reflection and is non-judgemental.

Supervision is partly about feelings and communication, but it is also rooted in considerations of clinical effectiveness or of evidence and best practice (Duff *et al.* 1997). It may include a discussion of how the practitioner felt in a particular consultation but it might also cover, for example, the right hypertensive treatment for the patient or the latest approach to screening for chlamydia. When the occasion requires, supervision can incorporate both technical and emotional knowledge, both scientific understanding and self-awareness.

Although most supervision consists of reflective conversations about active clinical cases – hence the term 'clinical supervision' – it can range more widely. It can involve reflection on past encounters that need mental or emotional processing, and it can also extend to reflection on other aspects of the practitioner's work, including interaction with colleagues (Bond and Holland 1998). We regard it as an important form of learning and we believe that in primary care the most useful definition of supervision is 'facilitated learning in relation to live practical issues'.

What do we mean by primary care?

The professions addressed in this book are mainly those connected in some way with general practice surgeries: GPs, practice nurses, health visitors, community nurses. Much in the book also applies to a wider circle of related professionals, such as community pharmacists and physiotherapists, counsellors and community mental health nurses. Some contributors refer to the supervision of mental health professionals, some of whom may be working within surgeries (for example, as attached psychologists and counsellors). However, we have intended the main emphasis to be on the needs of the 'front line' non-specialist practitioners working across the whole clinical spectrum rather than those who work mainly with internal mental health referrals. We hope that the book will be useful for any clinician working on the front line.

In the course of this book, some of the chapters address an interprofessional context, whereas others deal with only one discipline, such as general practice or nursing. Perhaps inevitably, much of the writing is about doctors. This reflects our own backgrounds as GPs and the fact that many of our colleagues from outside primary care first started their educational or supervisory work working with GPs. In addition, some of our arguments are derived from our research and our experience. The majority of our research has been based on doctors only, but not all of it. Our experience, again, is based mainly on accounts and interactions with doctors. But this is not exclusive and many of the vignettes and examples in these introductory chapters are from nurses, psychologists and others working in the community setting.

Another reason why the emphasis of this book is on GPs is that GPs as a professional group face an exceptional crisis of morale and identity. This crisis highlights the need for something like supervision. At the same time, the GP profession is far behind many others in thinking how to develop better survival mechanisms. We recognise that, in the changing world of a multiprofessional primary care service, research and work will in future be based more firmly across the different professional groups. We are also aware that doctors in particular may need to learn from many of the people they work alongside, especially nurses, who as a profession have collectively thought much harder about clinical supervision; and who as individuals may sometimes know far more about supervision than doctors.

Why does primary care need supervision and support?

Primary care, as a rule, is not characterised by the proverbial sore throats, dressings and ingrowing toenails that the public may imagine, nor by the relatively trivial function of 'gatekeeping' as understood by many specialists and politicians. It is a place of immeasurable complexity, uncertainty, unpredictability and muddle. It is also a place of refuge for those whose problems permanently defy definition, or who are too disturbed or frightened to go anywhere else. As an example, one GP provided us with the following sketch of six patients whom she saw in the course of a single morning surgery (personal details of cases, here and throughout the book, have been altered to prevent any possibility of identification).

Mrs A complained of feeling butterflies in her stomach the whole time. She denied any stresses of any kind, in her home life or at work. She just wanted to know why she always gets butterflies. Just as the consultation ended, she asked me if I could arrange plastic surgery on her chin because it is sagging – almost imperceptibly, as far I could see.

Ms B came in for a regular blood pressure check. As I put on the blood pressure cuff she asked if she could also have some antidepressants. On enquiry, it turned out she has lost both her parents in the past year and has no other contact with any living relatives. She says she has no idea how to find any meaning for herself in the future.

Mr C was a man with multiple sclerosis. Until now, he has always refused to let me tell his wife the diagnosis, pretending that it is a post-viral condition that will get better. On this occasion, his wife turned up with him and insisted I must tell her the truth. The patient said I must not, and then his wife said, in front of me: 'If you don't let the doctor tell me now, I'm leaving you.'

D was a teenage boy with back pain. The pain seemed trivial, but I asked him how he got it. He was abroad in Spain last week, on a school minibus that crashed. Two of his schoolmates were killed.

Mr E came in asking to be referred to a counsellor or psychologist. His wife has just fallen in love with someone else over the internet. She has asked him to leave the house and he has agreed to do so. He says: 'I still love her and I don't want to upset her.' Everyone he knows says he is mad, but he wants a counsellor or psychologist who will see his point of view. The couple have a handicapped toddler.

Mrs F came to have a regular blood test for her thyroid. As I was drawing blood she said can she ask my advice. Her niece has recently taken an overdose and following this has told my patient (but no one else) that she was sexually abused as a child. The niece has sworn my patient to secrecy, and she does not know what to do about this.

Many people outside primary care would listen to this account with incredulity, especially if they learnt that this list of patients was selected from among more than 40 that the doctor had seen in the course of one working day. They might assume that the doctor especially attracted these kinds of patients, or that her list was 'exceptional' in some way. But from our experience of talking to people within primary care, both nurses and doctors, the kind of caseload that this account reveals is commonplace.

Of course, the cases described above mostly concern problems that lie loosely within the area of mental health. Yet it would probably be an accurate assumption to expect that this doctor's workload on the same day, or any other day, would have included at least an equal number of cases where she had to make instant responses to similarly complex needs related to physical problems – or to problems that sprawled indefinably across a number of different areas, including preventive health, nutrition, benefits, housing, the law or immigration, to mention only a few. Some of these might have involved the use of interpreters or the presence of family members and other personal advocates. Other encounters, no doubt, related to cases where many other professionals played a part: colleagues within the same practice, the local pharmacist, hospital personnel, teachers and clergy . . . the list is limitless.

If any counsellor or psychotherapist were to see such cases, they would almost certainly think it worthwhile to seek some form of supervision on how to proceed. But most GPs and primary care nurses, together with all the other clinicians who work in primary care, have no such expectations. Huge numbers of interactions with patients take place rapidly, under pressure and with little or no time for reflection. Where supervision and support do occur in primary care, they may be haphazard and crisis-driven. Indeed, one could say that there is often a kind of 'inverse care law' at work here, whereby the professionals in our culture who actually see the largest number of people with complex and demanding problems, and have arguably the greatest need for supervision, have the least expectation of receiving any. It is also worth pointing out the paradox that it is exactly these kinds of cases, with their poignancy and human richness, that attract people to primary care in the first place and sustain them throughout their careers.

People with a mental health or social work background are often very surprised to learn that GPs, practice nurses, health visitors and other in primary care usually receive no case supervision. Primary care practitioners are often equally amazed to learn of this surprise. There is a contrast of ideologies, between the one which encourages reflection and institutionalises its use, and the one which has traditionally expected practitioners to cope with whatever arises from within their own resources – and which now faces external monitoring as the main driver for improvement.

Supervision and support in primary care: the current state of affairs

It would be unhelpful and also unfair to suggest that primary care is devoid of supervision and support. One of the things we have become aware of in our own work as educators is the very widespread and protean forms that this takes. In our experience, many practitioners say they receive little or no supervision and support because they think it only 'counts' if delivered in a formal manner. However, they can easily be prompted to recall encounters that arise on an almost daily basis when someone facilitates their learning in connection to practical work issues. Although they may not regard these occasions as supervision, they almost certainly qualify as such.

There are, for example, many practices where people talk to each other regularly about their day-to-day difficulties as they arise and may, indeed, drop in and out of each others' rooms or catch each other between consultations as a matter of routine. There are nursing and health visiting teams where practitioners on the ground feel supported by their peers and their seniors, and able to consult them on difficult cases. It is fairly normal nowadays for practices to hold regular team meetings to discuss problematical cases. Although some of these are about the exchange of information, many serve the same functions as clinical supervision. There are teams that sometimes carry out random case analysis or look at critical incidents or at opportunities for learning that may arise from encounters with patients (Eve 2000). A few teams may use attached mental health professionals, such as counsellors or therapists, for help in thinking about cases that are not actually referred (Deys, Dowling and Golding 1989; O'Reilly 2000). Many practices are involved in GP vocational training and this provides one model of how time may be structured within the working week for supervision and support. Case discussion happens there on a regular basis, both in the day-to-day interactions between registrars and trainers and on vocational training courses. It is fairly common for registrars to discuss whole surgeries, or certainly cases selected at random, at frequent intervals. A similar model is developing for an apprenticeship-based element in the training of nurse practitioners.

Beyond this, we have come across many educational and other approaches to continuing professional development that contain conspicuous elements of supervision and support even though they may be formally presented as something quite different, for example as postgraduate trainings, or as case discussion seminars. Much of this book is taken up with descriptions of particular approaches that we believe have clinical supervision and support at their core, and provide other models of the kinds of approach that might be developed or adapted on a much wider scale. Approaches like these offer home-grown or 'native' models of how primary care might introduce and develop a wider culture of clinical supervision and support. It is particularly important to notice and value all these kinds of supervision – and indeed to acknowledge the vast amount of effective 'self-supervision' that goes on inside the minds and feelings of many practitioners a great deal of the time. Many, if not most, practitioners carry out a constant process of self-enquiry and self-improvement – the 'internal supervisor'. Far from characterising primary care as a desert in terms of supervision, all these activities need to be noted and built upon. In promoting supervision, we feel it is important not to undermine the culture of primary care nor to dwell on its inadequacies, but rather to amplify what it does well in the normal course of its work.

At the same time, it is important not to lose sight of the enormous gap that exists between the amount and kind of provision that is generally available in primary care, and what is available or even mandatory in other spheres. While not oppressing people in primary care by emphasising their deprivations in terms of professional support, there is no reason to disguise the fact that people's expectations of supervision might be very much higher than they usually are – in regard to quantity, quality and the kind of patient care that might result. It is also important to acknowledge that there are some practices where even 'corridor conversations' are unknown because of isolation, fear, conflict, burn out or simply tradition. It is also important to note the dramatic cessation of supervision for many people working in primary care, in particular GPs, once formal training ends.

The obstacles to supervision and support in primary care

Given the difficulty of working in primary care, why is clinical supervision not already part of our culture there, in the way that it is with some other professions? In our researches, we have found that practitioners describe two factors as maintaining this state of affairs: workload and ethos.

Workload

Sheer workload is a constant complaint. These examples are from GPs.

> The scale of the work and the endlessness. The scale being that you go in at eight in the morning and be dealing with people's pain continually and without a break and go on to seven or eight in the evening: to a degree and with a volume that I think is almost inconceivable to most other outsiders. (West 2001)

> Even GPs with very even temperaments are working under a lot of pressure. We have so many things we have to do to earn our money ... We have to split ourselves in different directions, often with no supervision. So many GPs have nobody to help them develop appropriate coping strategies. (Reiss 1996)

Or, workload may be judged by the overwhelming influx of paper missives and pieces of information, the importance of some of which cannot be judged, as the total amount is unmanageable.

> You have ten tons of bumph coming through, fundholding, practice management ... you don't have time to read it all through ... (Burton 1996)

The influx of both paper and demand has increased exponentially in the last decade. Although the changes brought about by successive governments have created all kinds of opportunities for development in primary care, including much of the work described in this book, the experience on the ground has often been of persecution and of near collapse. Although one might expect that the very scale of workload might have led people in primary care to seek, even to demand, resources for reflection and support, it generally seems to have had the reverse effect. There has been a vicious circle whereby the scale of the problem has itself often overwhelmed the search for a solution.

As a result of this onslaught of clinical and organisational demands, many GPs tell of how they have learnt to cut themselves off from aspects of their work. They describe different mechanical ways of dealing with patients, such as delaying tactics – 'doing every test'. GPs themselves see some of their cut-off behaviour as fairly brutal – 'like a "callous surgeon"' – or simply as abrupt.

> Sometimes I close the door. There is no GP that doesn't do that unfortunately. We shouldn't have to, but we do. (Morris *et al.* 2001)

GPs have varying degrees of understanding of the defensive ways which they use in order to manage patients' illnesses and anxieties.

> The whole trade is to do with some very raw emotion. For that not to swamp us as an institution, we split all that off with the patients, and we keep the expert, calm reassuring side of the equation ... I think there is something deep and powerful in keeping illness and anxiety on the other side of the desk. (Reiss 1996)

Usually, doctors do not find it difficult to admit that help is needed, but may not know where to look for it.

> It is difficult I find not having anybody to go to with my problems who would give advice, who would be my tutor. Most people who do mental health work have a counsellor that they can discuss their problems with. I have no one. (Morris *et al.* 2001)

Ethos

One does not have to look far for accounts of primary care that make it abundantly clear that it can be a very unreflective work setting. These accounts implicate GPs in particular, and they possibly reflect wider cultural problems in the medical profession as a whole. Sometimes, they concern doctors behaving arbitrarily, and without any apparent sense of accountability, or connection with other agencies. Here is one example.

> A health visitor's assistant brought to a discussion group the case of a family. The children of this family were possibly at risk, as a result of the problems of one of the parents. She brought the problem to the group because, although she had tried many times to speak to the GP on the telephone, so that she could discuss the situation with him, he had refused to speak to her, and she didn't know what to do. The group too was distressed by the story and it was difficult to find anything to say, but, privately, group members who were GPs must have felt deeply embarrassed.

They must have looked into their memory banks to discover if and when they too had behaved like this, whether from stress, overwork, ignorance or plain arrogance.

People hear stories like this and comment on the 'pathology' of the primary care ethos. If they are managers, they may see events like this as evidence of system faults which either might be picked up by external monitoring systems or, in less severe situations, by internal monitoring systems – what is now called clinical governance. Another perspective is to view the problem as cultural and psychological: people identify the 'gung ho' culture of primary care, negative attitudes to reflection on problems and mistakes, and a widespread inability to admit weaknesses. We have quite often come across mental health professionals who see primary care as a 'sad' area, where standards of self-criticism and reflection are unacceptably low.

From an insider's perspective, things do not seem so simple. When primary care practitioners reflect on their own working experiences in protected settings, such as learning or support groups, they do not find it difficult to admit that they have many problems. But, because keeping going, appearing to cope and surviving are important and because there are no common routes to finding help, for many people these problems are never addressed.

The following kinds of comments about the ethos of primary care and its resistance to supervision are typical.

We have to be in control, in charge. Supervision carries with it a stigma of neediness.

There is a lot of fear around being judged as 'bad' or 'mad' or incompetent as a result of needing time to reflect.

Traditionally 'trained' doctors have not been thought of as requiring supervision.

Medical culture does not include it as a basic need. Cynicism and despondency are obvious and difficult to combat (Souster 2001).

Our own experience in many ways echoes these findings from research. In our work as educators, we hear regularly of practices and teams in primary care where reflective conversations are rare or non-existent. In some cases it is because practices have become dominated by the pursuit of technical or pragmatic ends, such as keeping to protocols or making profits. In these circumstances, people do not ask for supervision because they do not want it or because they believe – consciously or unconsciously – that it will interfere with their independence as experts or as business people. In addition, we hear of conflicts between GP partners, members of a nursing team, different professions within the workplace, or clinical and non-clinical staff. Largely, these may go undiscussed and unresolved. In primary care, there are no formal mechanisms to make sure that colleagues 'get on' in the interest of performing their collective task of looking after patients, and there are few facilities for obtaining help once this task has been impaired by repetitive infighting or even by communication effectively ceasing altogether. Sadly, we often talk to GPs and primary care nurses who say there is not enough trust within the team for members to expose their vulnerabilities or areas of ignorance. Nurses and other employed or 'attached' members of teams say that they, too, cannot easily enter into intelligent and non-judgemental case discussions because there is an assumption that they should just get on with their jobs, or because the sense of hierarchy within the primary care team inhibits them from asking questions or from offering help to colleagues who are 'above' them in the pecking order. Pharmacists and optometrists say that they are held back by the constant need to generate income and by the ethos of competition between practices.

Perhaps most worryingly, we hear of practitioners who become brutalised very early on in their careers in the health service, or who rapidly become disillusioned about their work and consider leaving it. Having entered their professions with idealism, they soon find that they cannot adequately hold on to compassion or curiosity once they meet with the onslaught of everyday work in primary care, often in conditions of professional isolation and unsupported by a sympathetic peer group. Untutored, they may adopt a cynical attitude, hardening themselves in order to cope with these difficult problems, in a way which has been discussed elsewhere by Marris (1996). The last thing they may think they need, let alone ask for, is time and space for reflection with colleagues.

Conclusion

In starting to think about the needs of any of the primary care professions for supervision and support, the volume and complexity of the workload, and the ethos, seem very daunting problems. If supervision is to be promoted within primary care, it needs to be done with a clear understanding of the scale of the need and the many forces that may lead to wariness, fear or resistance to the idea. There are a number of obvious questions to pose, including the following.

- How can one possibly seek or receive supervision on even a fraction of the cases or encounters in primary care where this might be beneficial?
- Is there any point in promoting supervision when most of the work will always have to be done in a more or less unreflective way?
- How can one introduce or develop a culture of clinical supervision without seeming to put yet another pressure or demand on practitioners?

We have no illusions about the huge challenges that these questions raise. We also have no simple answers. However, as an initial response to these questions, we want to propose three ideas.

1 Clinical supervision and support are not panaceas. They will always need to go alongside political and structural approaches that lessen the pressure on practitioners and make their lives more manageable.
2 Some supervision and support is better than none, and more is better than less – provided these are introduced in ways that are consonant with the realities of everyday work and ease the stress rather than turning the screw even tighter.
3 Once introduced, on however small a scale, supervision and support may have some effect on the overall culture in a team or a practice, and on its capacity to act reflectively.

Primary care clinicians have to deal, often without guidance, with an enormous, sustained and difficult workload. Clearly, the initial training of primary care professionals – either at basic or post-registration level – can never fully prepare them for their future professional duties. Studies show how practitioners may easily become brutalised and adopt mechanical working practices. Unreflectiveness can become institutionalised. We would like to identify our mission as challenging this unreflectiveness, where it occurs, and promoting cultural change so that it becomes less common. We see clinical supervision and support as a crucial part of such cultural change. We see them as forms of learning that fit best with the nature of the work in primary care, and with the needs of practitioners.

We know that some readers may feel that they receive almost no supervision and support, and we would want to encourage them to think about the first steps they might take in order to ameliorate that state of affairs. Equally, there will be others who feel embedded within existing systems for supervision and support; such readers might want to compare these systems with the ideas proposed in these pages or consider how they might disseminate resources to their colleagues more widely. We would also suggest that all practitioners, at whatever level, might benefit from considering the kinds of cases for which they currently get little or no supervision (including complex cases, stuck ones, cases that raise their anxiety and those where they feel they might have something to learn) and to think about how they might change this state of affairs.

References

Bond M and Holland S (1998) *Skills of Clinical Supervision for Nurses*. Open University Press, Buckingham.

Burton K (1996) *Child Protection Issues in General Practice: an action research project to improve interprofessional practice.* A report commissioned by South Essex Health Authority, Essex Social Services and the Essex Child Protection Committee. (www.londondeanery. ac.uk/gp/home.htm)

Deys C, Dowling E and Golding V (1989) Clinical psychology; a consultative approach in general practice. *J R Coll General Practitioners.* **39**: 342–4.

Duff L, Fennessey G and Harvey G (1997) Clinical effectiveness, embracing the challenges. Paper given at the National Board for Northern Ireland Annual Research Conference 'Research based practice: meeting the challenge'. In: Royal College of Nursing Institute (2000) *Realising Clinical Effectiveness and Clinical Governance through Clinical Supervision: Volume 4, The Reader.* Radcliffe Medical Press, Oxford.

Eve R (2000) Learning with PUNs and DENs – a method for determining educational needs and the evaluation of its use in primary care. *Education for General Practice.* **11**: 73–8.

Marris P (1996) *The Politics of Uncertainty – attachment in private and public life.* Routledge, London.

Morris P, Burton K, Reiss M and Burton J (2001) The difficult consultation. An action learning project about mental health issues in the consultation. *Education for General Practice.* **12**: 19–27.

O'Reilly J (2000) The practice as patient: working as a psychotherapist in general practice. *Psychoanal Psychother.* **14**: 253–66.

Reiss M (1996) *Evaluation of the Consultation Skills Course.* A report commissioned by North Thames East Deanery. (www.londondeanery.ac.uk/gp/home.htm)

Souster V (2001) *An Evaluation of the 'Working Models of Support and Supervision' Conference.* (www.londondeanery.ac.uk/gp/home.htm)

West L (2001) *Doctors on the Edge.* Free Association Books, London.

CHAPTER 2

The nature and purpose of supervision

Jonathan Burton and John Launer

We start this chapter with some accounts of supervision, describing what it involves – and what it does not involve. Following this, we look at some ideas about supervision from a number of fields, in particular the mental health world, and examine how these might be adapted for primary care.

What happens in clinical supervision?

Throughout this book, there are many examples of the kinds of problems that people bring to clinical supervision, and the ways they are helped. However, it may be useful at this point to give some brief descriptions of the kinds of encounter that we would regard as supervision. These descriptions are not meant to be normative or 'typical'. Clinical supervision can vary enormously according to the work setting, the time available, the nature of the problem, the needs of the clinician, the approach of the supervisor or team and so on. Nevertheless, we hope that these three accounts will give some sense of what we consider the territory of supervision to include.

> Ms B, a health visitor, was seeing a woman who caused her enormous concern because of how depressed she seemed. The woman came from Thailand, with no friends or relations in the UK. The husband was Scottish and 15 years older than his wife. They had only been married a year and they had just had twins. Ms B had a suspicion that the marriage had been arranged through an agency or perhaps just a classified advertisement. The wife seemed cowed by her husband, who clearly expected her to keep the house immaculate despite having two new babies. The husband seemed not to welcome Ms B's visits, and jokingly described his wife's

depression as 'playing for the sympathy vote'. Ms B asked to talk to her line manager about the case. The line manager spent nearly an hour with her exploring all the different issues in the case. These included the risks of serious puerperal depression, the demands of twins, the cultural and age differences between the parents, homesickness and isolation, and the difference in perceptions between the health visitor and the husband. Through the conversation, Ms B came to realise that she could make things worse by trying to 'rescue' the woman from her husband, and that she needed to build up his trust instead. She also came away from the discussion with a range of options in her mind. These included a joint visit with the GP, putting the mother in touch with the local twins' club, and exploring to see if there were any other Thai mothers in the locality who might be willing to make contact with the woman.

Dr A, a GP, was having a consultation with a patient in her early 40s who appeared to be having menopausal flushes, although she was still having periods intermittently. She was still taking the progesterone-only contraceptive pill and wanted to continue some form of contraception if there even was the tiniest risk of still being fertile. She was asking the GP if she could start on hormone replacement therapy (HRT) as well, although she was also concerned because her mother had died of breast cancer. She was hoping that HRT would help with her 'ratty' moods as well as flushes. Dr A felt unsure about what to advise because of the large number of different factors that needed to be taken into account. He asked the patient if he could leave her in the room for five minutes while he sought advice from one of his partners, who had recently been on a course covering treatment of the menopause. The colleague talked him through the various options he might offer the patient, including some that Dr A did not know about, such as the combination of oral oestrogen together with an intrauterine system delivering progesterone. She also brought him up to date on the issue of HRT and breast cancer risk, and reminded him to check if the patient smoked, as this would affect her range of choices. They both agreed that HRT alone might not make any difference to the 'ratty' moods, and Dr A would need to take up this theme with the patient as well.

Ms J, a clinical psychologist working in primary care, was seeing Jake, a 15-year-old boy, who had been referred because of disruptive behaviour at school. Ms J wanted to see Jake together with his mother, but for various reasons the mother always ended up leaving the boy alone with the psychologist. On the first occasion, the mother left a message at reception that she could not come in because she had an urgent dental appointment. On two further occasions she came into the room but brought in her three-year-old, who was so active that she had to take him out into the waiting room after a few minutes. Ms J knew that Jake's parents were divorced, his mother had remarried and the toddler was from her second marriage. Ms J therefore started to wonder if the boy's problems might be connected with his mother's difficulty in focusing on his needs – but was unsure how to make this point without seeming critical. She brought the case to the primary care team at their regular weekly case meeting. The team came up with a range of ideas. They suggested that Ms J could phone the mother at home to explain why it was important to have some protected time to think about Jake's problems, and to enquire whether there was a time that she could arrange child care for the toddler so that she could join Jake at the clinic. The team also helped her to think about the boy's relationship with his natural father and his stepfather, and how each might need to become involved in the meetings at some point.

These are the kinds of professional exchanges (among many other kinds) that we believe it is important to nurture and develop – or to establish where they do not yet exist.

What does not count as clinical supervision?

There are many legitimate and necessary activities in primary care that do not constitute clinical supervision, for example:

- training events that address facts, protocols, guidelines or management systems without looking at specific clinical cases
- meetings and conversations that involve exchanging information about patients, without any of the parties seeking to enlarge their understanding or to change their management of the cases
- encounters where the principal purpose is to carry out assessment or testing, or to take disciplinary action
- presentations and demonstrations of ideas and techniques where the recipients are more or less passive
- activities where the sole focus is on administration, audit, regulations or money.

In reality, however, some elements of clinical supervision may at times enter a whole range of activities, including those listed above, that did not set out to offer this. For example, a discussion about guidelines may well end up with practitioners citing particularly challenging cases – or types of case – and then exchanging ideas of how to manage these (or, alternatively, how to change the guidelines). Equally, a meeting about a formal complaint from a patient may well evolve into a group discussion of how to learn collectively from the event. For this reason, we believe it may not be helpful to regard any activity in primary care as absolutely excluding clinical supervision. It may be more important to look at how reflective conversations can become a more established part of everyday practice.

What is supervision for?

Brigid Proctor, who has been an influential writer in the field of clinical supervision, suggests that supervision has three purposes (Proctor 2001).

1   Normative: helping people to aspire to quality standards.
2   Formative: helping people in their professional development.
3   Restorative: offering people support in the difficulties they experience.

In Proctor's thinking, supervision is about empowerment. The sets of values and assumptions which underpin supervision include:

- a belief that practitioners are normally to be trusted to work well and to be self-monitoring
- a belief that reflection on experience and practice is a major resource
- a view that supervision is a co-operative exercise between people who share a common humanity and common professional interests.

Proctor's definitions of the purposes of supervision seem to be transferable to the primary care context, because they embrace the aims of quality of practice, professional development and support. We believe that, in today's primary care world, a working definition of supervision has to embrace all three aspects.

The normative aspect

There are many circumstances where supervisor and supervisee may work, more or less rigorously, to external standards of practice: for example, they may work to improve practice against an established evidence base, a recognised body of guidance concerning ways to conduct the consultation or in accordance with clinical effectiveness. The Royal College of Nursing Institute (RCNI) has recently sponsored a publication, for example, which is entitled: *Realising Clinical Effectiveness and Clinical Governance through Clinical Supervision* (RCNI 2000).

Alternatively, the supervision may occur in a setting in which standards of practice are uncovered or discovered during discussion: these standards may be called 'internal' standards. They may be less rigorous than external standards but they may be more realistic and acceptable, and therefore, in the real world, lead to greater change. For example, a facilitated group, looking at video-taped consultations, may establish its own internal standards for discussing the consultations. These standards may be based on what the group sees as the most effective way of helping each member of the group to build on their present level of expertise in the consultation.

If clinical supervision is not normative, it may be anarchic and ineffective. Poor performance and poor communication are rightly unacceptable. The revolution towards ever-improving quality is laudable. No one could argue that it should not occur. However, the normative aspect also carries inherent problems. Its immediate effect on individuals and teams, who are already feeling fully stretched, may be to create fear and defensiveness rather than a constructive response. Thus, the normative aspect needs to be balanced with other aspects – that nourish and sustain practitioners too.

The formative aspect

Carr (1995), an educationalist, writes that a key principle of being professional is that professionals ensure that their practice is constantly being re-interpreted and revised. This capacity for changing the tradition of practice is developed through what he calls 'critical reconstruction' of practice. Professionals, because they are professionals, are people who seek constantly to refine their practice. Throughout their careers they should be learning and refining their capacity to change.

In our interview-based evaluations and researches, we have established an extensive record of accounts of learning experiences. This confirms how vulnerable practitioners often feel, and how much they appreciate help with their difficulties. We take it for granted that most primary care professionals want to do well and, indeed, to do better. They constantly want to bridge the gap between what they are able to do and what they need to do. They would like to feel less uncomfortable and more confident about many of the things they do at work. Thus, one of the challenges of clinical supervision for primary care is to offer opportunities for a continual expansion of skills, competencies and understanding.

The supportive aspect

Raising standards and professional development need to take place in a supportive and non-competitive environment. Many writers appreciate that health professionals need and deserve support systems that recognise and value their important contribution, quite aside from any clinical or developmental aim (Morton-Cooper and Palmer 2000). Clinical supervision that is not intrinsically supportive is unlikely to be effective. One of the principal tasks of supervision is therefore to establish an atmosphere of positive encouragement and to promote a non-competitive culture in which people are motivated by praise and understanding rather than by criticism.

Supervision helps the supervisee to focus on resolving the 'here and now' difficulties of practice. It is one of the ways in which difficulties and puzzlement may be turned into opportunities for learning and improving practice. Taken altogether, it is a focused approach to professional development, involving the interplay of personal and professional experiences with the guidance of others in a supportive environment.

Supervision in the mental health professions

Many of the mental health professions recognise that patients are better-served if clinicians on the ground have career-long opportunities to keep the whole of their professional practice under constant review, and to discuss and learn from their everyday work experiences in a non-judgemental and reflective way. They also accept that practitioners are also likely to experience more job satisfaction as a result. In these professions, supervision is entirely distinct from any notion of education or appraisal. Instead, it is regarded as a non-judgemental but also essential means of achieving quality and professional development, and of providing emotional support for practitioners.

In mental health practice supervision is usually case-based and it is often undertaken between a senior practitioner (supervisor) and a less-experienced practitioner (supervisee). It may also take place in the form of regular multidisciplinary case discussions, for example by a weekly mental health team meeting. There will often be a defined methodology for supervision in these contexts, such as a standard way of presenting cases and being questioned about them. Because of the relatively small caseload these professionals have in numerical terms, it is often expected that every single case will be covered at some time in the course of supervision – something that would obviously be quite unrealistic in primary care. For some practitioners in these fields, it would certainly be unusual to carry cases, except for the most straightforward ones, that were never discussed at any stage with one of their peers. Far from seeming an irksome requirement, the opportunity to discuss a majority of clinical cases is usually valued as one of the most attractive aspects of this kind of work.

There are clear advantages to having a systematic approach in the way that some of the mental health professions do. Regular contact and case discussion with peers lessens the isolation that practitioners may feel and may lessen the risk of stress and burn out. The fact that supervision is entirely routine takes away any suggestion that it is primarily a policing activity. Although there are obviously instances where supervision uncovers real cause for concern about professional competence, these are relatively rare and therefore do not lessen the overall acceptability of supervision within the professional culture.

Practice in the caring professions generates intensely difficult feelings. Professionals may feel vulnerable not only in response to the difficulties of the work but also in the thought of exposing their difficulties. Regular supervision encourages an acceptance that this is so, and offers understanding and normalisation for what the practitioner is going through. Supervision may contain the fear of shame and discomfort, and can harness the capacity for creating and sustaining professional change. Giving a high profile to supervision pays acknowledgement to the seriousness and scale of the work done, and to the emotional difficulty and complexity of the work. It directly addresses the need to avoid emotional over-involvement (or under-involvement).

In the minds of many mental health professionals, there are other advantages too. Good case discussion may steer clinicians away from stereotypical or stigmatising descriptions of the people they are seeing, towards more compassionate and imaginative ways of viewing them. In this way, supervision can help to sustain ethical practice. In technical terms, supervision may help counsellors and therapists not to become ensnared in the content of patients' problems, and to look instead at the wider processes that are occurring, including the process of the therapeutic work itself. Indeed, supervision can itself model the way that people's problems can best be helped not so much by looking for solutions but by allowing these to emerge through dialogue and reflection. Supervision also models the way that different people can have entirely different perceptions of a situation, and a different repertoire of suggestions as to how to deal with it. It exposes people to the experience of discovering 'what they did not know that they did not know'. Team supervision, in particular, offers opportunities for different professionals working together to think how the same case might be addressed in different ways by practitioners coming into the discussion with different professions, ethnic backgrounds, genders or personal preferences.

Perhaps the most important advantage that regular supervision promotes is the acquisition of 'knowledge-in-context'. Facts and theories are not conveyed as abstract, disembodied information, but are derived from – and applied to – the authentic realities and shifting experiences of everyday work. Routine supervision encourages practitioners to enter a lifelong cycle of reflection and learning, in which knowledge, ideas and experiences continually nourish each other. Although supervision takes effectiveness seriously, it recognises that effectiveness is multiple and complex, and may involve more than the measurable. It invites reflection on what the clinical aims are, what means are being used to achieve those aims and what the evidence is for that. It promotes a less casual attitude to effectiveness primarily through meeting practitioners' needs – as a prerequisite to meeting those of patients.

Looking at primary care, it is clear there is a vast amount to be learnt from the way that supervision is regarded in these parallel professions – not least in the respect and priority accorded the professionals themselves in their need for reflective time and support. It offers them ideas to redress 'the inappropriateness and frustrations of reductionism' imposed on them by so much biomedical thinking (Butterworth 1992).

However, it may also be important for people in primary care to be aware of some of the limitations of supervision, and of the criticisms that have been made of it. Like any familiar activity, supervision may become stale and repetitive. It may encourage practitioners to institutionalise conservative forms of practice because neither they nor their supervisors challenge working practices that have become comfortable and easy for everyone involved (Feltham 2000). Supervisors and supervisees can fail to get on, or may get on well but collaborate unwittingly in the joint pursuit of inertia or poor management. Neither party can necessarily protect the other against overwork, professional brutalisation or personal illness and loss. Supervision can 'become an arena for anxious case management rather than for reflective understanding' (Woodhouse and Pengelly 1991). It can also become theory-driven or dominated by organisational needs, or it can turn into an inappropriate form of personal counselling (Northcott 1998). Supervision, in other words, is not a panacea.

The psychotherapeutic approach to supervision

In much of the literature on supervision, writers recommend similar kinds of technical approach, including the use of open questions, exploring options and offering suggestions for consideration (Tichen and Binnie 1995). Many of the techniques suggested involve the sort of facilitating behaviour that is common in person-centred counselling. However, the field of psychotherapy offers a particular approach that requires a separate and more detailed discussion here – in particular because some of the writers in this book base their chapters on it.

Much supervision within the field of psychotherapy focuses on the feelings of the practitioner as the main source of information regarding the patient and the nature of the patient's problem. This is based on a belief that patients always 'transfer' their habitual patterns of dysfunctional behaviour, or their negative expectations, into their relationships with the professionals they meet. According to psychotherapeutic understanding, this stirs up reciprocal feelings (for example, of anger, pity or sexual attraction) in the professionals themselves: hence the terms 'transference' and 'counter-transference'. Supervision in psychotherapy very often involves careful reflection on the therapist's responses to the patient, and an analysis of how and why the patient has provoked these. This may include considerations of how relationships with important figures in the therapist's own life – in particular parents – may also be playing a part in what is going on in the consulting room. Most psychotherapists and some other mental professionals argue, or simply assume, that this kind of work is the basis of all effective clinical supervision.

The potential of this kind of approach for revealing crucial information about the patient and about the therapeutic process is enormous. Its applicability to primary care is also easy to see, for example in helping practitioners to think about patients who consult in a seemingly perpetual spirit of disappointment, bitterness, reproach, flattery or flirtatiousness.

However, this approach too has its own particular limitations. It demands a very great deal of time, and a relationship of great trust between practitioner and supervisor. It is also based on the assumption that both parties have had personal psychotherapy themselves, allowing them to develop a particular kind of sensitivity when observing their own reactions, and an ability to tolerate someone else commenting on these in detail. Without all these precautions in place – and even sometimes with them – there is a risk that supervisors may launch into inept and damaging interpretations of what is going on, and supervisees can feel exposed or humiliated as a result.

Adapting these approaches for primary care

In thinking about how to adopt or adapt these ideas for primary care, a number of factors need to be considered. Most obviously, the workload for all the primary care professions is numerically much vaster than in counselling or therapy, and the pressure of time is much more intense. Also, although many problems in primary care are 'pure' mental health ones, most include aspects where factual biomedical knowledge and technical expertise are as important as interpersonal skill and emotional sensitivity. Many of the problems we see in primary care are essentially 'seamless' ones, sprawling across the boundaries between clinical, managerial and organisational domains. None of these aspects of the work is less important than the other. Because of this, different approaches to supervision may be needed at different times, or by different people. Some are more likely to want to concentrate on the difficulties of relationships with patients, colleagues and self, whereas others are keen on the discussion of clinical and organisational matters. For primary care, the challenge is how to acknowledge the affective or psychosocial dimensions of encounters with patients and colleagues without losing touch with the practical side of the job, or straying into areas that are potentially too disturbing for practitioners.

In this connection, it is worth noting that many apparently 'technical' or bio-medical exchanges between practitioners are probably already closer to forms of supervision in mental health and even psychotherapy than the practitioners themselves may realise. Typical examples of this are where one GP asks another for a second opinion on an ECG, or when a practice nurse seeks advice about how to respond to a patient's poor results on their peak flow or blood sugar record. Although the requests seem superficially to be factual ones, they are often framed within a brief narrative that actually provides a wealth of information about the patient and the consultation too. (For example: *'This ECG has been brought along by a chap of about 20. His anxiety is sky high although his symptoms don't amount to much. Unfortunately the ECG isn't quite normal and his dad has some sort of heart disease. What do you think I should do?'*) The consequent conversations, even if highly condensed, may have many of the characteristics of more formal supervision of the kind practised in psychotherapy, including the intensity of focus, the seriousness of the reflection involved and the important part played by contextualisation. The brevity of the encounter may, in fact, belie a tremendous sophistication of thought, especially if the practitioners are highly experienced, know each other well and share a working language.

At the same time, there is another factor to be considered. Many primary care practitioners, by necessity, need to 'fly by the seat of their pants' for much of the time, without consulting anyone, and perhaps using tried and tested strategies without a great deal of conscious reflection, but there is no clear evidence that this is a bad thing. Requiring practitioners to be constantly self-critical, or to make greater efforts to sustain emotional contact with the suffering they encounter, has risks as well as advantages. The apparently casual, unreflective, sociable way in which many primary care encounters take place may seem to some observers to be open to criticism, but it may also have merits. The general practice consultation, for example, represents a mode of interaction that is socially sanctioned and may serve an important ritual and narrative function in many people's lives. It is by no means clear that replacing it with something much more scrutinised, self-conscious or explicitly therapeutic in style would be welcome or, indeed, any more effective. There may sometimes be advantages to 'not thinking' in primary care.

Related to this is the question of how safe it is for primary care practitioners to expose themselves emotionally to the full scale of the distress they encounter in their work. It is certainly possible to argue that good psychological defences are necessary in order to survive the scale and pace of work. The main challenge might not be the need to notice the transference in each individual consultation, but to survive in the face of a daily avalanche of human distress. Much of our work in primary care may be mentally unprocessed, at least in the way that other professionals might consider desirable, but it may not be less effective as a result. Many of the problems we see remain unresolved and perhaps irresolvable, but primary care may fulfil an important social role as a place for such problems to be brought, and part of the practitioner's role may be to tolerate this without a sense of inadequacy and failure. Indeed, one task for supervisors might be to consider how risky it would be for practitioners to become too intensely involved in reflection, and therefore to lose their tolerance of 'stuckness', their spontaneity, their humour or other culturally appropriate and useful attributes, including the capacity to be rude when the occasion requires it.

In considering what can be transferred from one culture to the other, there clearly needs to be a balance. On the one hand, people in primary care need to acknowledge the different working practices, constraints and beliefs that operate in their work settings. They need to be conscious of the impossibility of introducing supervision 'across the board' and of the need to be selective in the cases – or the types of cases – where they seek help. On the other hand, they might benefit greatly from an understanding of the way that other professions look after themselves in organised and respectful ways. In the end, however, the synthesis will need to be one that feels consistent with the work itself. To quote Brigid Proctor again:

> Health practitioners – and indeed each group of professionals – need to develop supervision training, models and skills which are immediately useful and practicable in their own context. (Proctor 2001)

How effective is clinical supervision?

There is no point promoting any activity like clinical supervision unless it can be shown to be effective. We now address its effectiveness.

Models of clinical supervision, both from within primary care and from parallel professions, show how it can resist unreflectiveness and help to maintain a culture of enquiry, curiosity and change. There is a plethora of evidence from case experience and from the collective development of whole professions that shows the benefits of supervision (RCNI 2000). Our own evaluations of many courses and conferences related to supervision and support amply support our personal impression that these things are often received 'like rain in the desert', and help to revitalise people's professional commitment (Souster 2001). From evaluations carried out by some of the contributors to this book (Hiew and Sivananthan 2002), it is clear that practitioners within primary care also feel sustained and revitalised by activities involving supervision and support. In qualitative studies of such activities, these kinds of comments are extremely common:

> It diminishes your sense of failure with what is a classic heartsink sort of patient. We have all got patients like that and they all leave the consulting room leaving us feeling very drained ... And to be able to show how you

coped with a patient like that for the scrutiny of your peers, is actually very reassuring. (Reiss 1996)

I feel validated in the difficulties I have. I understand more of the system I am part of. I have stopped being too responsible. (Launer and Lindsey 1997)

Such studies provide very many individual accounts of rejuvenation. They also provide strong prima facie support for the idea that wider introduction of clinical supervision and support might help to address widespread problems of demoralisation in primary care, as well as issues of recruitment and retention.

However, these studies have their limitations. We do not know, for example, whether supervision increases the statistical chance of practitioners in any field staying in their jobs. We do not have any independent studies informing us if supervision actually enhances clinical performance, or whether it has measurable benefits on patients themselves. Nor do we know how the many individuals who at present do not have supervision are able to develop their own strategies for sustaining morale and competence.

There is clearly a large research agenda here. If clinical supervision is to be taken seriously in primary care, we will need to pay attention to evaluation as have other professions. We will need to show how time invested in supervision is rewarded – either by time saved in other ways or by improvements in performance, or in workforce patterns. Some possible research questions might include the following.

- Can regular clinical supervision prove itself to be cost-efficient by helping practitioners to meet the needs of frequent consulters more effectively, and therefore to lessen their consulting rates?
- Can the rate of referrals to mental health services be lessened through a programme of supervision aimed at supporting professionals in maintaining patients in the community?
- Could a practice improve its rating on standard measures such as the Consultation Quality Index or Patient Enablement Instrument (Howie *et al.* 1998; Howie *et al.* 2000) by a regular input of supervision?
- Can a programme of clinical supervision reverse trends of early retirement and poor job retention, or attract more people who want flexible working patterns?
- Can clinical supervision help individuals prepare themselves for the periodic inspections that are now in place for appraisal and re-accreditation – or to pursue the directions that may be indicated by these inspections?

Perhaps the most important question for the future is what constitutes 'enough' supervision and support for primary care. In other words, input might be required to ensure that practitioners in different situations remain competent, enthusiastic, reflective and continuously capable of learning in their work. Answering questions like these will not be easy and we are likely to need more sophisticated research approaches than many current ones.

Conclusion

Clearly, there are many concepts and approaches from other fields that can provide primary care with a starting point in thinking about the nature of clinical supervision, its purpose, its uses and its effectiveness. Some of these concepts and approaches may be readily transferable, but many would not, or would need considerable adaptation. As part of the health and social services, we are probably at the point where we need to start examining how we might move the culture of primary care towards a position where we have our own established ideas and ways of practising supervision.

References

Butterworth T (1992) Clinical supervision as an emerging idea in nursing. In: T Butterworth and J Faugier (eds) *Clinical Supervision and Mentorship in Nursing.* Stanley Thornes, Cheltenham.

Carr W (1995) What is an educational practice? In: *For Education: towards critical educational inquiry.* Open University Press, Buckingham.

Feltham C (2000) Counselling supervision: baselines, problems and possibilities. In: B Lawton and C Feltham (eds) *Taking Supervision Forward – enquiries and trends in counselling and psychotherapy.* Sage, London.

Hiew S and Sivananthan N (2002) The partnership for progress in practice project. *J Learning Workplace.* **3**: 6–10. (www.tlw.org.uk)

Howie J, Heaney DJ, Maxwell M and Walker J (1998) A comparison of a patient enablement instrument (PEI) against two established satisfaction scales as an outcome measure of primary care consultations. *Family Practice.* **15**: 165–71.

Howie J, Heaney DJ, Maxwell M and Walker J (2000) Developing a 'consultation quality index' (CQI) for use in general practice. *Family Practice.* **17**: 455–61.

Launer J and Lindsey C (1997) Training for systemic general practice: a new approach from the Tavistock Clinic. *Br J Gen Pract.* **47**: 453–6.

Morton-Cooper A and Palmer A (2000) *Mentorship, Preceptorship and Clinical Supervision.* London, Blackwell.

Northcott N (1998) The development of guidelines on clinical supervision in clinical practice settings. In: V Bishop (ed.) *Clinical Supervision in Practice.* MacMillan, Basingstoke.

Proctor B (2001) Training for the supervision alliance attitude, skills and intention In: J Cutliffe, T Butterworth and B Proctor (eds) *Fundamental Themes in Clinical Supervision.* Routledge, London.

Reiss M (1996) *Evaluation of the Consultation Skills Course.* A report commissioned by North Thames East Deanery. (www.londondeanery.ac.uk/gp/home.htm)

Royal College of Nursing Institute (2000) *Realising Clinical Effectiveness and Clinical Governance through Clinical Supervision.* Radcliffe Medical Press, Oxford.

Souster V (2001) *An Evaluation of the 'Working Models of Support and Supervision' Conference.* (www.londondeanery.ac.uk/gp/home.htm)

Tichen A and Binnie A (1995) The art of clinical supervision. *J Clin Nurs.* **4**: 327–34.

Woodhouse D and Pengelly P (1991) *Anxiety and the Dynamics of Collaboration.* Aberdeen University Press, Newcastle.

CHAPTER 3

Raising the profile of supervision and support in primary care

Jonathan Burton and John Launer

A constant theme of this book is that supervision cannot be seen as one single concrete method or approach that is entirely distinguishable from everything else. In this chapter, we want to propose that the most effective way of raising the profile of supervision and support in primary care may be to see it as an aspect of many different activities that already happen in primary care, and to promote it as such. Following on from the argument of the previous two chapters, we believe this may have several advantages:

- it builds on what already exists and is familiar in primary care
- it recognises the particular needs of primary care, including the constant need to integrate technical knowledge into case management
- it connotes supervision as something natural and necessary, rather than something special and perhaps a bit 'precious'.

Supervision as an aspect of education and training

There is an unarguable case that some form of technical learning should happen throughout the professional life cycle (for example, learning about new drugs, research evidence or treatment protocols). Virtually everyone working in primary care now attends some form of education, whether in the form of attendance at postgraduate lectures, short courses or practice presentations by colleagues or drug representatives. However, it is clear that much of this learning is disconnected from the active contexts – the cases – in which it will always need to be applied. The abstract principles of the protocol or formulary may only make sense when fitted to patients' experiences, beliefs and needs. This can only be learnt through reflection on specific cases.

The Oxford dictionary defines education as being 'a form of instruction in preparation for the work of life'. We have carried out a great deal of research into the perception held by GPs and practice nurses about their past and present education. Many of those we have interviewed have felt that their earlier education has failed to prepare them for what they end up having to do in the primary care setting. Their mainly hospital-based training has not fitted them for the world of primary care. One nurse, for example, described how she had felt *'Absolutely shocked ... and out of my depth completely'* in her first week working in general practice. For GPs their earlier education has not only failed to prepare them for the workload and strains of general practice, but frequently it has also been abusive or frightening. This is especially true in the early stages.

> The education we get as doctors is quite intimidating. There is a lot of ridicule if you don't get it right. It is not a useful way to learn. (Reiss 1996)

> The medical students on the ward who were then known as ward clerks had imposed on them the duty of doing all the blood-taking, because they were a cheap pair of hands. I went up to the bed with this blood-taking kit, and this chap lay there *in extremis*. He had the diagnosis of multiple myeloma, which meant nothing to me at that stage. As I approached the bed, he turned one eye towards me and said: *'Go away boy, can't you see I am dying?'* And that was my introduction to clinical care. (Reiss 1996)

Even during their time as junior doctors in hospital, some interviewees remembered feeling that they were under-helped, and that they were just made to absorb the culture of 'grit your teeth and get on with it'.

> Nobody talked to us about how to cope with the job or how to help the parents or how to be with these dying children. Or how to cope with your own feelings. You were expected to cope, so you cut yourself off in a way. (Reiss 1996)

In specific areas, too, GPs reported that they were under-prepared. For example, in respect of child protection issues, a GP who took part in an action learning project remembered, as a student, going to a child protection case conference.

> It gave me some idea of the issues involved and the different agencies and how they related to each other. It was almost as if they were in a different

world, one I couldn't understand. I don't know. It was something I had never come across in my upbringing. (Burton 1996)

Another GP reported:

In medical school we didn't really have a lot of contact with patients directly who had been abused. I can't remember a specific scenario we were involved in. Obviously we had lectures on it, but I don't really have any first hand experience. I suppose it was information you just assimilate. Really much of what you take in at university is basically to get you through an exam. (Burton 1996)

In some way things are now changing, with more emphasis on community-based teaching of medical students and better preparatory training for practice nurses. Many GPs make up ground during their period of vocational training and especially from their attachment to their GP trainer. A similar form of apprenticeship for practice nurses who are training to become nurse practitioners, with a one-to-one relationship with a professional mentor at work, is arising at present. This, too, will provide a form of induction into the work of primary care. Despite this, however, there is still a widespread sense that the emphasis, content and ethos of much training at both pre-registration and post-registration level is still unhelpful in the sense that it does not prepare people for the work they actually do. There is also a perception, widely supported by research, that an unhelpful ethos continues to influence formal professional education. Seemingly, much education even at the level of continuing professional development is still too divorced from the actual realities of daily working life (Boud 2001). The work of the Innovations in Education Research Group (IERG) (*see* Preface) included interviews involving more than 100 health professionals. The same reflection came up time and again: early education does not adequately equip them for a significant part of their work. In their descriptions of their problems, respondents seemed to be acutely aware of the contrast between the fact that they are 'highly educated' but basically 'unprepared'.

In fact, education and clinical supervision need not be seen as entirely separate. Instead, one could see supervision as an indispensable aspect of the educational process. It is possible to incorporate elements of technical training into a framework of supervision, or to make space for the discussion of specific cases as a way of testing the validity and applicability of abstract knowledge, such as guidelines. Either way, we would argue that decontextualised learning should no longer be seen as a higher priority than learning from reflecting on cases. Instead, it might perhaps be better to conceptualise clinical supervision as an indispensable aspect of learning for practitioners who have to face the complex and indefinable realities of their work, as opposed to the sanitised abstractions of the lecture room, journal article or textbook. This is consistent with Schon's

(1983) conception of the 'reflective practitioner', who is capable of learning in context and of reflection in action.

How might this work? Readers will find examples at several places in this book of ways that different clinicians and educators have found to 'square the circle' between technical learning and case supervision. Here, we draw attention to just two of these. In Chapter 10, Jonathan Burton, Steve Hiew and Nalliah Sivananthan describe the self-directed learning movement. They describe how groups of primary care professionals used a form of collaborative enquiry to learn in the peer group setting. Actual encounters with patients were the learning material. Commitment to the principles of clinical governance was written into the rules of the group. The authors show how peer supervision has the capacity to improve technical performance – by harnessing new knowledge, skills or attitudes to working performance. Writing about this experience elsewhere, Hiew and Sivananthan have shown that group members aspired to emulate the professional practice of their peers – a good example of the normative aspect of supervision. Measurable improvements in the care of groups of patients had been achieved (Hiew and Sivananthan 2002).

Similarly, in Chapter 12, John Launer looks at how clinical supervision might become the mainstay of GP vocational training. He suggests that clinical supervision can take account of many other necessary aspects of the trainer's task, including assessment and pastoral care as well as education. He puts the case that it may be useful 'to think of clinical supervision as lying at the core of vocational training, and to see the other aspects of training as modifying it but ideally not displacing it'. Readers may want to consider whether this idea might also work in relation to the approaches described in some of the other chapters too. In other words, it may be helpful to regard all the various contributions in this book as pointers to how the focus of many educational activities in primary care might be moved towards case-based supervision as opposed to more abstract forms of learning.

Appraisal and its dilemmas

In the last few years, appraisal of health professionals has taken off with extraordinary speed, and has acquired irresistible momentum. Whilst writing this book, we have seen it introduced into the discipline of general practice. Indeed, while putting the finishing touches to this book, we were aware that many details of the GP appraisal process were still unclear and that there was some abiding ambiguity about its nature and purpose. We therefore offer the following comments in the almost certain knowledge that the situation will develop further by the time that readers come to consider them.

In theory, appraisal is a formal and imposed monitoring process designed mainly to ensure that the individual is practising to accepted standards. Appraisal is therefore linked to a preset external agenda and to general standards, rather than to clinicians' specific needs in relation to the events of their everyday work, although it is also meant to encourage the process of further professional development (GMC 2000; ScHARR 2002). The General Medical Council (GMC) has suggested that the process of appraisal should cover the seven items of good medical practice.

1 Good professional practice: working within the limits of their competence; not putting patients at risk.
2 Maintaining good medical practice: keeping up-to-date and maintaining skills.
3 Relationships with patients.
4 Working with colleagues.
5 Teaching and training.
6 Probity.
7 Health.

GP appraisal in Britain has been greatly influenced by a report from the School of Health and Related Research at the University of Sheffield (ScHARR 2002). This report emphasises appraisal as a way of improving practice across the spectrum. The following is ScHARR's definition of appraisal:

It is a positive, developmental, employer-led, two-way, action-oriented process, primarily directed at quality improvement.

However, the report (ScHARR 2002) recognises that appraisal will need to be a collaborative enterprise rather than an imposed one:

In the present context of general practice appraisal will not be welcomed by some, but it will be difficult or impossible to implement effectively without the co-operation of GPs.

In other words, there is clearly a tension at the heart of appraisal. On the one hand, it is designed as an external driver to improve quality. On the other, it is also conceptualised as a collaborative, peer-led activity.

Despite the emphasis placed on development and collaboration, it is perhaps understandable that appraisal in primary care causes much anxiety among GPs. This anxiety is shared both by appraisers and those to be appraised. Partly, this is because of concern that there may sometimes be a need to carry out 'policing' or to take disciplinary action as a result of appraisal. There is also concern that appraisal is part of a wider project to steer primary care practitioners in the direction of public policy, rather to address their personal developmental needs. Despite the use of words such as *development*, there is a widely held expectancy that the process may end up feeling uncomfortable and threatening. As we write, it is unclear whether there will be minimum standards by which appraisees may be judged. However, appraisal will certainly demand a new sort of relationship between an appraising colleague and the appraisee. The reality is that a commitment to the intention to change is more or less imposed under a formal contract.

The appraisal system for GPs is to be based on personal development plans (PDPs). There are some specific concerns in relation to these too. One of these is the tension between individuals' needs and those of the practice, locality or nation. Another concern is about the relevance of PDPs. They may not address many issues of performance beyond those that are easily quantifiable. Certainly, PDPs are not likely to address core skills such as how to re-orient practitioners towards asking open questions, coping with the unpredictable, addressing complexity. They may not achieve one of their prime tasks – encouraging practitioners to uncover what they 'did not know that they did not know'. PDPs may well include, for example, a demonstration that a practitioner has attended an 'update' on the treatment of asthma. But a PDP cannot demonstrate that the practitioner can adequately manage an encounter with a patient who is reluctant to use a steroid inhaler, or who puts pressure on the practitioner to over-prescribe oral steroids.

Can appraisal and professional development go hand-in-hand successfully? There are arguments to suggest that this may be difficult, and that there is a case to be made for separating appraisal of GPs from their professional development. Others argue, however, that the two processes should always be joined together (Northcott 1998). We do not have easy answers, and there may not be any. However, from our perspective as primary care educators and as advocates of clinical supervision, we would offer the following ideas.

- There is clearly a need for all the professions, and for the managers and politicians who regulate them, to balance the external and compulsory processes, such as monitoring, with the fostering of internal and elective processes, such as clinical supervision. The former may possibly be capable of addressing serious under-performance. It is almost certainly only the latter that can address the kind of professional development which enables people to link their knowledge and skills to actual practice, and to deal with complexity, indeterminacy and the uncategorisable muddle of everyday work.
- If there is to be an overview of professional standards in order to detect and eradicate poor performance, that overview should examine established markers of good practice (GMC 2000). It is possible that this may be better

conducted by external analysis of data (for example, the quality of referrals and the number or type of hospital admissions) than by peer interview.

- Over a professional lifetime, most change probably occurs by chance and in response to events. It is cumulative and occurs on many fronts at once. Personal and professional change are intimately linked, and relatively little change occurs by explicit intention. Experience-based learning of the kind promoted by clinical supervision may therefore be more effective over the course of a career than prescribed or negotiated learning of the kind that appraisal may require.

- No one should underestimate how much any encounter between professionals may be affected by a difference in power between the parties involved. Although it is perfectly possible for someone with more power (for example, a trainer or employer) to act supportively and non-judgementally, the person on the receiving end will always be aware of being vulnerable, and may alter what he or she says or does as a result.

- The adult learning model assumes that the learner is learning as a free and self-determining adult (even if within a system of rules and regulations) (Brookfield 1986). In other words, he or she needs to be able to say: '*I know that I work within a system of rules and regulations, which I accept. But I want my own competence as a learner to thrive, so I need to maintain a large degree of personal control over my learning.*' The adult professional, going through a repeated exercise of appraisal, will therefore need to have a significant level of control over the process, and to feel some mastery over the experience of being reviewed.

Supervision: an essential complement to appraisal?

It is worth noting that the Department of Health (DoH) has made an explicit commitment to promoting clinical supervision:

> It is central to the process of learning and to the expansion of the scope of practice and should be seen as the means for encouraging self-assessment and analytic and reflective skills. (NHS Executive 1993)

It is also worth noting that PDPs were originally introduced in the context of promoting continuing professional development, and only later harnessed to formal appraisal systems. Although there has been a shift in the last few years to a preoccupation with 'risk avoidance' rather than 'fostering excellence', the door has not yet been closed on parallel approaches to professional development that are based on voluntary, collective and professionally appropriate methods.

In some medical specialities, the two already run side by side. Child psych-iatrists, for example, take part in annual appraisals and are obliged to keep PDPs, but for most of them this is a comparative formality, since nearly all of them are engaged in regular case discussions on at least a weekly basis with other members of the mental health team (as well as doing joint clinical work with some of them).

If the primary care professions can overcome the feeling that they have been taken over by external political processes, they may be able to demonstrate that clinical supervision can help to address public anxieties about competence, and even to meet government objectives effectively. Although there will always be a need for adequate systems of monitoring and discipline for the professions, it may still be possible to demonstrate to managers and politicians that it is more intelligent, and more effective, to invest in 'half-full bottles' than to investigate 'half-empty' ones. As Souster (2001) writes:

> Effective and well managed supervision and a positive attitude to profes-sional support play a major role in the clinical governance agenda. This is particularly pertinent to risk reduction strategies in general practice set-tings, where many individuals work in isolation and have no professional support. There is a need for local leaders to empower primary care staff, so that support and supervision are embedded in working life as an indispens-able tool, helping people to deal with the problems and challenges of everyday working life.

Another way of looking at this might be to encourage a different view of 'fitness to practise': one that views fitness not in terms of jumping over fixed hurdles, but in terms of being able to fit the working environment – and to develop that kind of 'fit-tingness' as a continually evolving process.

If this is to happen, the primary care professions will themselves need to take the initiative in introducing forms of supervision that are effective in raising standards and that are seen to be effective. But there are also ways that super-vision and appraisal could work together, particularly if the judgemental aspect of appraisal can be kept within acceptable boundaries or hived off into a separ-ate, external process.

One way that supervision and appraisal might work together would be to equip appraisers with the skills needed for clinical supervision. This is not to sug-gest that appraisers should spend their time supervising appraisees on specific clinical cases. Rather, such skills might assist the task of being an appraiser by helping to establish a more facilitative style of appraisal interview. Through acquiring such skills, appraisers might also develop a greater understanding of the styles of learning appropriate for primary care, and might therefore come to a more sophisticated understanding of what personal development involves for adult practitioners. Similarly, those about to be appraised might find it helpful to prepare themselves for this experience by being in a supportive relationship – with an individual or within a group – to help in the preparation for appraisal. After an appraisal, individuals might find it helpful to take back to a group or colleague the kinds of tasks that now appear to lie before them. It might therefore be helpful for appraisers to be linked into local networks, such as self-directed learning groups, so that they can point people in appropriate directions for such support. Developing this kind of linkage between appraisal and supervision could potentially be a effective way for primary care organisations to disseminate a culture of clinical supervision around their districts.

Conclusions

For most clinicians in primary care, there is a large and constantly expanding base of knowledge to be mastered, and performance to be maintained, but we believe it is an error to conceptualise this task as a disembodied bundle of facts that is separate from the day-to-day experience of cases and must be learnt only through traditional methods. Conceptualising learning and development in this way may, in fact, impair sensible application of knowledge, or even appropriate recollection of it. We see clinical supervision as covering a continuum of activities that can sometimes run alongside the facilitation of learning and can sometimes be entirely separate from it. Because practitioners have to change constantly, and in many ways, they need to use a variety of methods to do so. Some learning can indeed occur either through doses of formal educational or through the gradual personal learning that helps the steady adjustment of competence through life. Some may occur as a result of appraisal. However, we promote the benefits of supervision because it deals with 'here and now' problems in the way that no other approach can offer, and because it can help practitioners to become aware of what they were not aware of before. We do not advocate clinical supervision as an exclusive approach to learning, but we do argue that, for all primary care practitioners, it is an essential part of learning that now needs to be pursued and evaluated with vigour.

We want to ask our colleagues in primary care to consider how they might demonstrate the effectiveness of supervision and support, and therefore challenge managers and politicians to question current assumptions underlying the funding for such activities – or the lack of it. Readers might also want to think about their own local circumstances, and about how to make credible claims for resources so that they can raise the profile of clinical supervision among their colleagues generally.

We would like to invite educators to consider how clinical supervision might be put at the centre of training and appraisal activity at the different levels: from pre-registration training, through post-registration training and then right through professional life as part of lifelong learning. This book concentrates mainly but not exclusively on the different parts of a GP's career, but the accounts set out and the lessons drawn can probably be applied generically to all professionals working in primary care. Another issue is how supervision might be protected – both structurally and philosophically – from the plethora of regulations, curriculum demands and other bureaucratic requirements imposed by outside structures. Above all, we want to suggest that the time is now ripe to think about how we might all promote a culture of clinical supervision and support for all the professions in primary care.

References

Boud D (2001) Knowledge at work. In: D Boud and N Solomon (eds) *Work-based Learning. A new higher education*. Open University Press, Buckingham.

Brookfield S (1986) Understanding how adults learn. In: *Understanding and Facilitating Adult Learning*. Open University Press, Buckingham.

Burton K (1996) *Child Protection Issues in General Practice: an action research project to improve interprofessional practice*. A report commissioned by South Essex Health Authority, Essex Social Services and the Essex Child Protection Committee. (www.londondeanery.ac.uk/gp/home.htm)

General Medical Council (2000) *Revalidating Doctors. Ensuring Standards. Securing the Future*. General Medical Council, London.

Hiew S and Sivananthan N (2002) The partnership for progress in practice project. *J Learning Workplace*. **3**: 6–10. (www.tlw.org.uk)

NHS Executive (1993) *A Vision for the Future: the nursing, midwifery and health visiting contribution to health care*. HMSO, London.

Northcott N (1998) The development of guidelines on clinical supervision in clinical practice settings. In: V Bishop (ed.) *Clinical Supervision in Practice*. MacMillan, Basingstoke.

Reiss M (1996) *Evaluation of the Consultation Skills Course*. A report commissioned by North Thames East Deanery. (www.londondeanery.ac.uk/gp/home.htm)

School of Health and Related Research (2002) *Appraisal for GPs: executive summary*. (www.doh.gov.uk/pricare/gpappraisalexecsumm.pdf)

Schon D (1983) *The Reflective Practitioner: how professionals think in action*. Temple Smith, London.

Souster V (2001) *An Evaluation of the 'Working Models of Support and Supervision' Conference*. (www.londondeanery.ac.uk/gp/home.htm)

PART II

Perspectives from mental health

CHAPTER 4

Supervision in psychotherapy and counselling: a critical space for learning

Helen West and Linden West

Introduction

We work as teachers and researchers in higher education as well as psychotherapists. We share an interest in exploring the boundaries between learning and healthcare, and in processes of subjective and emotional learning in the professional development of healthcare workers and educators. We have experience of supervision in educational contexts, including supervising research students and trainees in guidance and careers education as well as of being supervised in psychotherapy. Our perceptions, for present purposes, have been specifically shaped by direct experience of supervision within psychoanalytical psychotherapy training and post-registration contexts, as well as an engagement with the now extensive literature on the subject (for example, Lawton and Feltham 2000; Scaife 2001; Shipton 1997).

This chapter draws on our experience of diverse supervision and supervisors, included in our training, post-registration work in doctors' surgeries and in other community-based specialist mental health locations. We want to share some thoughts, based on this experience, about the nature and purpose of supervision and relate these to the debate about supervision for primary care professionals, especially doctors. In the process, the various functions supervision may serve and the qualities needed for a good relationship between supervisor and supervisee are examined. We emphasise, as do the editors in the introduction to this volume, the common humanity, rather than hierarchy or surveillance, which needs to characterise supervision if it is to be meaningful and of real benefit for everyone involved.

Our experience of supervisors and different kinds of supervision is varied. Not all our experience of supervision or of supervisors has been easy, which is unsurprising. Like therapists and doctors, supervisors vary, as do the emotional dynamics that characterise relationships. We have struggled with particular supervisors, yet in retrospect, even difficult and painful encounters can enable us to make more sense of our work, including the unconscious processes in supervision itself. These include transference and counter-transference dynamics, in which a supervisor may be experienced as an omnipotent, omniscient parent, who knows, or ought to know, everything. In turn, we may feel stupid, ignorant, crass and inhibited. It is important to be sensitive to what we bring to supervision, negative as well as positive; conscious and unconscious. Psychotherapeutic training is rigorous at exposing the mixed motives and dynamics that are inherent in all human relationships. For instance, we may be envious of a supervisor and his or her knowledge and experience; this envy, derived from our sense of inadequacy, may inhibit the potential of the work.

It should be added that, in the main, our experience of supervision and supervisors has been positive. In writing the chapter and sharing our stories we were reminded, time and time again, of supervisors who challenged and confronted, but in empathic, learning-orientated ways. Working as a therapist, like being a GP, can be deeply satisfying, but it also raises troubling, often disturbing issues when engaging with patients whose life experience may be too terrifying even to name. The distinguished psychoanalyst Michael Balint once famously observed that working with disturbance disturbs. Patients' emotional problems and suffering affect therapists (as they do doctors or nurses) in diverse, unpredictable, often unconscious ways. Meaninglessness, pain, abuse and suffering in patients' stories may touch raw experiential nerves in therapists and lead them to ask questions about the value of their own lives, and the meaning and resolution of difficult experience within life. Like many doctors, therapists are often motivated towards their profession because of difficulties in their own life histories. Therapists (like the GPs to whom Balint was actually referring) have to learn how to manage and learn from disturbance, including their own, and supervision provides an important space in which to do this. Orbach (2001) has written that how we feel in our bodies, the passion or the ennui that is stimulated by our work, may be as important for learning as are the blood pressure cuff, the thermometer, the swab, the urine analysis, the X-ray and the ECG for doctors. Such feelings can provide a royal road to deeper levels of understanding about human interaction, the inner world of the patient as well as our own.

In this chapter, we wish to define some of the key functions of supervision in psychotherapy before exploring particular experiences of supervision, by reference to case study material (altered to ensure anonymity but maintaining, we believe, its poignancy). We devised a composite case study, drawing on our work with a number of patients to illuminate how supervision may serve different functions.

On supervision and its functions

Most definitions of supervision focus on the idea of a professional relationship that aims to help the therapist and the client to achieve better client outcomes. For example Edwards (cited in Shipton 1997) suggests that:

> the word supervision is generally used to describe the process by which a therapist or trainee receives support and guidance in order to ensure that the needs of the client are understood and responded to appropriately.

The challenge, of course, is to translate such general aspirations into a meaningful reality. In seeking to achieve this, supervision is often seen to have a tripartite function: monitoring, supporting and facilitating therapists' development (Lawton and Feltham 2000). These three functions suggest three roles for the supervisor: manager, counsellor and teacher. Inskipp and Proctor use a similar schema (described in Scaife 2001). Inskipp and Proctor refer to: the normative dimension of supervision (to induct the therapist into the standards and culture of the profession); the formative (to develop the therapist's skills, understanding and capacities); and the restorative (to address the tensions of the work and enable the therapist to continue to work for the best interests of the client without succumbing to burn out).

These three overlapping functions may be summarised as follows.

- Monitoring: concerned with ensuring standards and best practice.
- Learning: focusing on the development of clinical skills and associated theoretical insights, but also the development of self-understanding.
- Supportive: including focusing on, containing and processing the patient's emotional impact on the therapist.

The weight ascribed to each of these functions will partly reflect the values and needs of the professional context, the stage or needs of therapists, and the orientation and professional role of the supervisor. It may be argued that the last two functions overlap considerably; without support, for instance, there can be little learning, other than in the most perfunctory of ways. And monitoring, if conducted empathically, can be positive and reassuring in developing as therapists. There may be a danger in an NHS culture – where trust may be diminishing – of losing sight of some of the potential benefits of monitoring, in the sense of critically engaging with what we do in a developmental way in the light of widely accepted professional and service standards.

The monitoring function

The monitoring function is important, if problematic. Of course, mixing line management with supervision can be deeply counter-productive. If a supervisor is also a line manager, this can lead to conflict about how open therapists really can be, particularly in relation to possible mistakes or errors of judgement. Psychotherapy and counselling in the NHS context may be affected, like other forms of provision, by a blame culture, with negative consequences for professional development and relationships.

Moreover, as a number of commentators such as Feltham (2000) remind us, when viewed sociologically, supervision may be a system designed to 'keep counsellors in order' and to impress 'on the public that serious steps are taken to monitor and preserve quality' at a time of widespread insistence on professional accountability. Feltham (2000) also questions the implications of mandatory supervision, suggesting that it makes it difficult for therapists to be open about their experience, especially their mistakes. The experience of supervision can sometimes, he suggests, be redolent of school, evoking negative connotations of being checked on, and placing a premium on 'getting it right'. But this is to take an overly negative view of supervision: good supervision transcends many tensions and part of the supervisor's task is to encourage reflection on the supervisory experience and what may inhibit or facilitate critical learning.

We also emphasise the positive dimensions of monitoring in relation to our work. Initially, the supervisor can be crucial in inducting a trainee therapist into the norms and conventions of the discipline and professional culture, as well as into the particularities of the sub-cultural contexts in which a therapist might work, such as a GP surgery, where knowledge of professional hierarchies may be crucial to successful practice (Scaife 2001). Moreover, to use management language, supervision can be central to the quality assurance systems of a service, for new and experienced therapists alike. The baseline – given that the supervisor has some responsibility for patient welfare (Scaife 2001) – is to ensure that therapists practise in an ethical, safe and competent manner. That is important, not the least for therapists as they struggle, in the early stages, with complex issues, including ethical questions, and whether they might be doing more harm than good. However, effective supervision involves much more than this.

The learning function

A core role for supervision is clearly to facilitate the development of the knowledge, skills and attitudes necessary for therapists to function effectively and reflexively with clients. Lawton and Feltham (2000) outline the value of supervision for trainees and beginners:

> Supervision is probably the main place where real, vivid learning and discovery happens . . . where theory and reality meet in the challenge of actual

clients and the idiosyncratic demands they make on counsellors. The opportunity and the need to de-brief, discuss and reflect on and anticipate next steps in clinical work are usually keenly appreciated.

We concur with this interpretation and have keenly appreciated supervision when dealing with difficult, demanding patients, as our case study will make clear. Supervisor and therapist engage in a number of different but interrelated processes under the banner of learning. One encompasses the theory–practice dialectic, enabling theory to be informed by the nuance of the patient's story, much as a doctor needs to locate the technical and scientific aspects of medicine within a patient's wider narrative. Therapists need to learn to be flexible in relation to theoretical or clinical standpoints, to use different approaches with different clients, while adhering to some core principles of practice, such as the appropriate use of empathy, the development of a working alliance and the maintenance of boundaries. Therapists may begin to feel more confident in the quality of their work as they gain a more nuanced and a flexible perspective on a patient, by use of ideas and clinical techniques as servants of therapy rather than its master. Therapists also have to learn to remain 'human' in their work and not to detach themselves from patients by objectifying them and giving them a convenient but ultimately reductive 'label'.

The term 'critical learning' is used to encompass what is of central importance in supervision, which requires some definition. By 'critical', we mean, as Stephen Brookfield has written, an open, honest and imaginative engagement with experience in all its dimensions, which enables us to break through to new ways of seeing and acting in the world (Brookfield 1987). Being critical implies a way of being in the world rather than an abstract quality; it acknowledges the limitations of what we know, and can ever know, and our need for others in the business of lifelong learning (West 2001). It encompasses different ways of knowing, including emotional insight as well as intellectual, a critical knowledge of self, and self in action, as well as theory (Brockbank and McGill 1998).

The supportive function

Supportive relationships are a prerequisite of learning. Supportive supervision may enable therapists to better understand, and use therapeutically, their own reactions to patients, however disturbing. It helps therapists to contain and process some of the distress and messiness that may characterise particular encounters. It emphasises the human – not superhuman – nature of therapeutic work. Supervision, by fostering an attitude of 'curiosity' in all concerned (patient, therapist and supervisor), helps therapists to move beyond their own 'blocks', such as irritation with a patient for not making 'progress', or a sense of inadequacy in themselves. Importantly, an attitude of curiosity helps to keep therapeutic work 'alive' and therapists motivated, particularly at difficult stages of therapy, or when the work environment, for instance in primary care, proves frustrating.

There are countless moments when feelings evoked in therapists have to do with their own emotional and relational histories, as much as those of patients. Some therapists, for instance, may feel uncomfortable working with patients with eating disorders if that has also been an issue for them. Therapists have to be able to acknowledge such feelings and think critically with their supervisor about them, which, in turn, can enable therapists to regain a more empathic connection to the patient. Patients' disturbance and needs can only be met properly by a therapist functioning 'well enough', who is aware, or capable of becoming aware, of his or her own vulnerabilities as well as strengths. On occasion, therapists concentrate only on patients' problems and neglect their own. This may serve to avoid their own disturbance rather than learning from it.

Although supervision is not therapy for therapists, there are nonetheless parallels between the work of therapists with clients and the work of supervisors with therapists. One of the main tasks for therapists, for instance, is to build a therapeutic or working alliance with their patients, to enable them to be active participants in therapy, to gain understanding of themselves, their situation and of how, and why, to change. The purpose of psychotherapy, at least in its more analytical modes, is the struggle for understanding, meaning and personal responsibility, rather than more mechanistic forms of 'treatment'. Similarly, in supervision, supervisors and therapists need a working alliance to enable them to address issues together, in the search for meaning, insight and effective practice. Although therapists have 'hunches' and sense where a patient may be going, the important task is to understand *with* the patient. Similarly, supervisor and therapist have to work towards *joint* understanding, with supervisors being alongside therapists, rather than, over-judgementally, acting from on high.

Detachment

However, it is not quite that simple. Successful supervision also requires a sense of detachment in the supervisor. If supervisors stand alongside us in an experience, they have also to stand back and ask in an empathic way some difficult questions, including looking critically at therapists' possible misreadings, oversights or prejudices, as therapists do with their patients. Supervision can enable therapists to stand back more confidently in their own right and appreciate more of the processes that were not necessarily obvious in the session, to digest and 'metabolise' how a patient was experienced in a session and their reaction to this. Effective therapy requires therapists to maintain a fine balance between empathic understanding of patients in their situation, including being absorbed in their worlds, while distancing themselves from that world in order to think critically about what might be happening, including in their own emotional lives. Good supervision mirrors good therapy, being open to experience while providing some distance and detachment.

A case in point

At this stage, we use some clinical material to illuminate more of our argument. The case study below illustrates how the various functions of supervision may work in practice, in the interests of patients as well as therapists.

Working with patients who evoke anti-therapeutic feelings in therapists

The case study is derived from therapeutic work with a number of male and female patients in NHS psychotherapy departments and GP surgeries. Stephanie is not a real patient; she is derived from our experiences of working with a number of patients and her story encompasses real experience and illuminates how supervision can provide an essential space for critical learning.

We often find working with patients who harm themselves a particular challenge because they evoke such a range of feelings in us. We can feel fearful for the patient's safety, and angry with the patient for 'causing' us to feel fearful, manipulated, powerless and dependent. We have sometimes experienced a kind of hostile dependence at the heart of a relationship as part of a patient's deliberate sadistic strategy, which can, in turn, evoke the desire to retaliate. The anger we can feel emanates, in part, from the frustration with what seems to be an intractable situation, including the patient's resistance to an 'empathic' approach. The patient wants us to be there but not in the way we want to be, that is, empathically and with a commitment to change. We can struggle with the strength of the patient's pathological attachment to self-harming behaviour. Supervision can help us to work therapeutically despite own strong feelings and the urge simply to tell the patient, on occasions, to stop the behaviour 'for goodness sake'.

> Stephanie is 28 and married with no children. She was referred for therapy to deal with depression and relationship problems at work. She explained in the first session, with some hesitation, that she felt people at work gossiped about her behind her back and thought she was 'odd' in some way.

This so upset her that she 'went sick' and could not face work. She spoke quietly in sessions and looked away for most of the time. It did not feel as if this was a result of being shy, rather that Stephanie was holding something back, having a kind of secret, which she 'knew' the therapist might want to know. She acted in tantalising ways in each session, suggesting a possibility that all would be revealed. This evoked feelings of apprehension in the therapist (what was this terrible secret?), as well as of frustration and anger at her holding back. Stephanie felt distant and yet close at the same time, as though she could see the therapist's vulnerabilities and play on them. It was difficult to establish any kind of working alliance.

Stephanie's early history emerged only gradually in her narrative. She had, she would say, a caring childhood though one beset by a range of minor health problems, such as food intolerances and intense sibling jealousy. She felt she was different from her brothers and sisters who were much more straightforward and did not face the problems she had to contend with. Her relationship with her parents was deeply ambivalent, and she alternated in her narrative between being very positive about the happiness of her childhood while being angry about how uncomfortable it had been for her. Her view of herself was perpetually contradictory: she wanted to be different and yet did not want people to say she was different. It was proving impossible for the therapist to understand how she saw herself as different, and the extent to which this related to her secret. As the therapist felt closer to understanding her story, this would change, however slightly, and the therapist would feel as far away as ever. She intimated that she had had a special relationship with her father but it was not clear what this was or how she felt about it.

Stephanie had begun to cut herself in her teens as exams and decisions about what do to on leaving school approached. Cutting gave her relief, she said, as her 'secret' gradually unfolded. Her parents found out and were very angry with her. On one occasion a friend took her to hospital where she was treated for the wound and given some counselling. As she settled into work after school, a series of jobs in different retail outlets, she stopped cutting so much and was able to get on, a little better, with her life. She was married at 24 and now, at 28, had to cope with new changes. Her husband, who was in the services, had been promoted and they were due to move to another area of the country in a few months' time. She started waking early in the morning and thought about hurting herself for much of the time. The therapist was bothered by the amount of time and energy invested in the thoughts of harming herself. This seemed as bad as the actual physical harm she did to herself.

The information emerged over a number of sessions and with difficulty. Stephanie continued to look down to the floor much of the time and in one session began to fiddle with a little nail file, pushing it, first casually and then more determinedly, into the palm of her hand. The therapist commented on what she was doing while Stephanie continued to play with the file. There was a sadistic quality to the moment. Eventually, the therapist got her to put the nail file on the table, although the process was repeated on a number of occasions, as she kept picking the file up. Stephanie was always insistent about the importance of the sessions and said she could not function without them. She would occasionally telephone or leave letters for the therapist at the clinic. The therapist, in turn, felt angry at this clinging dependence as well as considerable discomfort in particular sessions.

Stephanie's case was discussed regularly in supervision, which enabled the therapist to continue to see her and maintain a therapeutic stance. The therapist was deeply reassured by the fact that the supervisor was monitoring the work. The 'quality assurance' dimension provided feelings of 'safety' as well as providing a wider perspective. The supervisor had been responsible for many psychotherapists and counsellors. There was a confidence that he could help the therapist assess what was being done from a broad basis of knowledge of different kinds of patients, therapists and therapeutic approaches. Equally, his professional and human insights and experience – his palpable humanity combined with a capacity for analytic detachment – meant the therapist could be open about the anger, frustration and destructive feelings provoked by the patient. Each time the therapist talked about Stephanie there was a sense of relief. The therapist felt 'refreshed' because of not feeling 'alone' with such a patient's intense disturbance and neediness. It was as though the therapist could 're-group', enabling the resentment and the struggle to cope with perpetual demands to subside. The therapist felt more resilient and 'professional' in contrast to the feelings of being embattled, even bewildered, in the early stages of the work. Supervision also engaged with more theoretical issues, drawing on a broad literature, but this was done in ways that emphasised Stephanie as a whole person to be thought about and understood in her own right, rather than a problem to be objectified. A degree of normality and balance was restored to the process. Supervision enabled the therapist to resist the seductiveness of the 'secret story' and to work with it. Without supervision the therapist could well have closed off from the patient and ended the work prematurely.

Supervision was important in other ways. Supervision helped the therapist to consider the strength of the patient's attachment to her pathological behaviour, and the extent to which she could experience suggestions of change as threatening to a way of being in the world which had at least enabled her to survive, however precariously. Supervision also encouraged deeper engagement with the literature and research on how patients who harm themselves frequently mention the relief they gain from such actions. An appreciation of wider evidence, and a deepening understanding of one particular person and her troubled story, brought the whole issue of self-harm, and appropriate therapeutic responses, to life in a dynamic way: experiential and conceptual learning, mind and heart, supervisor and supervisee and, to an increasing extent, patient and therapist, working in closer harmony.

The therapist was also learning about self. Acknowledging the power of the impulse to hit back against what was experienced as the patient's hostile dependence was an important step, as was to admit that the therapist often wanted to scream, '*Put down that nail file, it is driving me mad!*' This therapist needed to stand back and think of other ways of managing the disturbance, of what might help to establish more of an alliance, including drawing on the 'adult' side of Stephanie '*Could you put that down now please as it is a distraction to both of us*', delivered assertively but empathically, was one phrase that worked. Discussing highly practical techniques alongside the theory mattered greatly, as did involving other professionals in the case, thus broadening the basis of support for the patient and, incidentally, for the therapist as well. Contact was made, for example, with Stephanie's GP, and the therapist and doctor came to support each other in caring for her. She was also encouraged to consider a range of support services, including The Samaritans and the out-of-hours psychiatric services, if matters got out of hand at the wrong time. Stephanie had been reluctant to use other services but the therapist felt more confident as she became aware of the resources available, if needed, in the darkest moments. Obviously, the question of confidentiality in relation to talking to the GP was addressed from the outset.

Stephanie has stopped cutting herself and continues to make progress.

Supervision and learning

George Bernard Shaw once remarked that you can ask the most difficult question or make the most challenging of observations, if done in the right way – like the 'composite' supervisor mentioned above, who embodied the normative, formative and restorative requirements of supervision in a dynamic and sensitive way. The quality of relationship was crucial in creating an environment in which challenging questions could be asked. If therapists distrust their supervisor or feel criticised in a negative way – and this can happen – a relationship is likely to be stilted and unproductive. Therapists can feel alone in their work and may be unable to relate to it more analytically. Anxiety in therapists, if unresolved, may undermine the therapeutic process. Good supervisors, on the other hand, help to create an environment in which therapists feel 'safe' enough to engage fully with learning, in all its potential messiness and uncertainty (Mollon 1997).

Scaife and Walsh (2001) provide a useful summary of some of these ideas. They, too, equate effective supervision with a culture of learning in which the main emphasis is on positive thinking and openness to feelings, rather than negative evaluation and judgementalism. Good supervision explicitly acknowledges:

- the personal effect of work with patients
- the influence of events outside therapists' work on encounters with patients, including the location of the therapy
- the influence of the personal life history, values, beliefs and characteristics of therapists in working with patients.

If these are recognised as legitimate subjects for supervision, and assuming degrees of maturity, self-knowledge and sensitivity in supervisors, therapists can work with the anger, inadequacy or even boredom which all therapists feel from time to time in their relationships with patients.

Staying human

Supervision is becoming more rather than less important in the overstretched, increasingly frenetic atmosphere of healthcare provision that affects psychotherapy and counselling provision too. Therapists are not immune from the pressure of numbers or of accountability and evidence-based practice. Therapy, like a GP's surgery, is constantly in danger of becoming like the proverbial production line, given a broad range of clients, an increasingly explicit accountability framework and ever-growing demands in a context of stretched and stressed human resources. NHS therapists and counsellors inhabit, in the editors' words, a 'real world' too, having to balance the needs of patients with available resources and the ethos of an organisation. In such contexts and times, patients may become yet another demand; especially when they fail to fit a neat allocation of service resources or available therapeutic packages. At such times, supervision helps us all to stay human.

Conclusion

Good supervision, we have suggested, encourages forms of curiosity and reflectiveness that are neither intrusive nor prurient. It enables therapists to think creatively as well as critically about patients as individuals for whom experiences and feelings have particular meanings. The process can invigorate therapeutic work as well as motivate and re-invigorate therapists, when times get hard – as they inevitably do. On the basis of what we know experientially about the role of supervision in psychotherapy, and also from research into the struggles of doctors, we are convinced that supervision can support doctors in dealing with the complex, often uncertain demands of their patients and thus avoiding some of the burn out and low morale which currently bedevils the profession (Salinsky and Sackin 2000; West 2001). This can happen whether the context is a Balint group or more informal relationships with colleagues.

These are big issues since the subjective and emotional dimensions of primary care continue to be neglected. Supervision can help professionals to contain and process the disturbance that often and invariably surrounds their work. The neglect of the emotional and human dimensions of being a doctor, for instance, may be getting worse in a hard-pressed and even abusive system. Writing, for instance, about the impact of greater accountability and weeding out the unacceptable in medical practice, Salinsky and Sackin (2000) conclude that the focus on interpersonal and emotional issues in medicine, such as those surrounding the doctor–patient relationship, is in danger of going to the bottom of the pile, whereas 'the archaic system of junior doctor training in medical schools means that many students become less person-centred and lose their humanitarian ideals'. Such a conclusion is deeply worrying.

We have also argued that critical learning lies at the heart of meaningful supervision and that such learning requires a supportive and containing relational framework. This is learning which encompasses self, self in action, as well as the more theoretical and clinical dimensions of being a therapist. We have emphasised, too, that the ability to remain curious in the light of disturbance and confusion often requires regular supervision on a recurrent basis, and not simply in the early stages of working as a therapist. Therapists, like doctors, get tired and lost. They also need to feel restored. A sense of common humanity, as well as detachment, in a supervisor can enable experienced as well as new therapists to interrogate difficult, muddled moments, and to question the taken-for-granted, when it matters. Therapists are taught to be sensitive to their own needs, and to seek support as part of their ethical responsibilities. Such a requirement is needed across primary care.

Our ideas of critical learning also challenge the emphasis given to the 'independent' self-directed adult learner, as emphasised in some of the literature on GP education (West 2001). Instead, we want to stress the notion of interdependence rather than independence in learning. Learning is, at its core, a profoundly inter-subjective experience, in which we need others and supportive relationships at all stages of life. Research into adult learning reveals how 'significant others' are frequently crucial to progression in life, in particular at times of stress, major change and uncertainty (West 1996; West 2001). We exist, and learn, in a shared space of affective intercourse, in which there is a fundamental overlapping between one and another (Diamond 1998). If we feel accepted and legitimate we become open to learning in all its dimensions: to the play of the imagination; to new thoughts; to our feelings, however scary; and to the possibility of new directions in our work. Supervisors can play the role of the good-enough, significant other, creating a transitional space for learning, which can make a real difference in the struggle we all share between professional growth or atrophy, openness to new experience or defensiveness, professional health or 'dis-ease'.

References

Brockbank A and McGill I (1998) *Facilitating Reflective Learning in Higher Education.* Open University Press, Buckingham.

Brookfield S (1987) *Developing Critical Thinkers: challenging adults to explore alternative ways of thinking and acting.* Open University Press, Milton Keynes.

Diamond N (1998) On Bowlby's legacy. In: M Marrone (ed.) *Attachment and Interaction.* Jessica Kingsley, London.

Feltham C (2000) Counselling supervision: baselines, problems and possibilities. In: B Lawton and C Feltham (eds) *Taking Supervision Forward – enquiries and trends in counselling and psychotherapy.* Sage, London.

Lawton B and Feltham C (2000) *Taking Supervision Forward – enquiries and trends in counselling and psychotherapy.* Sage, London.

Mollon P (1997) Supervision as a place for facilitating thinking. In: G Shipton (ed.) *Supervision of Psychotherapy and Counselling – making a place to think.* Open University Press, Buckingham.

Orbach S (2001) Is there a place for emotional literacy in the learning environment? *Counselling and Psychotherapy Journal.* **April:** 4–7.

Salinsky J and Sackin P (2000) *What Are You Feeling Doctor? Identifying and avoiding defensive patterns in the consultation.* Radcliffe Medical Press, Oxford.

Scaife J (2001) *Supervision in the Mental Health Professions – a practitioner's guide.* Brunner–Routledge, Hove.

Scaife J and Walsh S (2001) The emotional climate of work and the development of self. In: J Scaife (ed.) *Supervision in the Mental Health Professions – a practitioner's guide.* Brunner–Routledge, Hove.

Shipton G (ed.) (1997) *Supervision of Psychotherapy and Counselling – making a place to think.* Open University Press, Buckingham.

West L (1996) *Beyond Fragments: adults, motivation and higher education.* Taylor & Francis, London.

West L (2001) *Doctors on the Edge: general practitioners, health and learning in the inner-city.* Free Association Books, London.

CHAPTER 5

Supervision in primary care: support or persecution?

Andrew Cooper

Trust

When I am supervising I think hard about what I am hearing, and when I think hard I tend to frown. During a review of our supervision, a supervisee said to me, '*You frown a lot while I am talking, and it makes me feel that you are critical of what I am saying*'. This chapter proposes that good, regular supervision is essential to the organisation of effective health and mental health services in the community, but also that it is as much a skilled and delicate undertaking for those receiving supervision as for those providing it. This is so because the supervisory process requires us to expose our practice to others, and this inevitably makes us feel vulnerable. There is little point in only rehearsing our successes in supervision, because one of the main objectives of practice supervision is the development and improvement of the service we offer. Some models of professional supervision emphasise this aim almost to the exclusion of another – the professional development of the individual practitioner. The kind of supervision discussed in this chapter places the day-to-day working experience of the practitioner at the heart of the supervisory process. Supervision is about *learning from experience* and, as in all walks of life, this feels like a risky and uncertain undertaking. In turn, this means that trust in a supervisor is an essential prerequisite of a meaningful supervisory relationship.

In the exchange described above, it emerged that my supervisee did not entirely trust me because she feared I was thinking critical thoughts about her work. But, how is it possible to engage in a process of true learning from experience without some element of critical self-reflection? One of the weaknesses of the conventional model of the 'reflective practitioner' is that it usually fails to engage with this delicate question, which is always lurking at the core of the supervisory experience. We all have a capacity for self-criticism, but this can take a more or less helpful form, depending upon whether it is a spur to self-examination and reorientation of our thinking about ourselves, or self-immolation and despair about our own worthlessness. Probably most of us fluctuate between these positions in relation to our experience of our own work. Recognising all of this, it becomes clear that the job of the supervisor is to constitute the supervisory relationship as a space in which supervisees feel safe to explore their practice experience without risk of feeling any more judged, persecuted or criticised than they are already liable to do by virtue of their own internal self-critical faculties. In a political and policy climate where 'governance' and 'accountability' become easily confused with the blaming and shaming of allegedly 'failing' institutions and their staff, such a model of supervision can sound almost subversive.

Everyday anxieties

Ordinary working life for primary care health and mental health practitioners brings them into daily contact with a continual stream of anxieties, fears and mental pain carried by patients and service users. Practitioners may appropriately think of themselves as having a rather defined or specialised role in patients' care, but from an emotional standpoint patients may not function in a fashion that is at all congruent with this expectation. Sometimes a seemingly ordinary and uncomplicated consultation leaves us feeling depressed and perturbed, or a patient to whom we think we have been helpful suddenly attacks or rejects us; a particular user leaves us feeling uncharacteristically incompetent, or we find ourselves feeling unusually angry and punitive towards a patient. These experiences are common, but equally they usually catch us by surprise and throw us off balance in our work. These are simple examples of the complexity of emotional experience in ordinary practice, but they point the way to the need for supervision which can help us to understand what is happening and, on the basis of this understanding, find ways of modifying our interaction with patients which may, in turn, be helpful to them. A common myth about supervision is that it is only needed in the context of specialised forms of work, such as counselling or mental health. In fact, wherever staff are in contact with patients – wherever there is some form of *relationship* at work – then difficult emotional transactions will be found. One of the best discussions of the value of supervision in primary care settings is by Dilys Daws (1995), who writes about her work providing supervision and consultation in a busy inner city health centre. She describes her monthly meeting with the group of health visitors:

> We will talk about a case that is perplexing them or, even more likely, irritating them or angering them. We talk about where these feelings come from, about how some people provoke anger and rejection as they go

through life. In particular, vulnerable new parents may elicit in a receptive health visitor feelings that really belong within unresolved relationships with the parents' own parents. Spotting this process may help health visitors to manage it. Wryly seeing that their feeling that they have somehow 'got it wrong' for the mother connects with the mother's experience of not being supported by her own mother and can make a big difference to their tolerance of it. Because the health visitor does then not snap back at her, the mother may then start to feel understood and supported at a crucial emotional moment in her life ... Feeling supported herself, the mother in turn manages her own baby's feelings better. When this happens, there is a wonderful chain of people getting things just a bit better than they have done previously, with a better start in life for a baby.

Dilys Daws' mention of the 'receptive' health visitor introduces an important new consideration. In order to make thoughtful and effective use of emotional experiences of the kind we have been discussing, practitioners must themselves be emotionally receptive. But this is a double-edged matter. Being receptive to the mental pain and emotional turmoil of service users entails us experiencing some of this turbulence and anxiety in our own right. Bluntly, *good* primary care practice will often be emotionally testing and confusing for the worker. A worker or even a team of practitioners who are impervious to the emotional dimension of their practice are not only cut off from their patients' struggles and dilemmas, but they are probably storing up trouble in other ways – an escalation of violent or threatening behaviour from users, or perhaps a high rate of staff turnover because of burn out.

Emotional exhaustion: good or bad?

There is a paradox here, illustrated by the following account of a small research study. As part of a larger evaluation of the impact of a consultancy project in a social services department, the researchers administered a well-known questionnaire designed to measure the emotional state of staff in welfare organisations. Some scored high on 'emotional exhaustion' and supposed 'burn out', some medium and some low. The researchers brought together three groups of staff who shared these different ratings and asked them to respond to a case study as though they were the social work team responsible for the situation. Those whose scores indicated low burn out responded in the least creative and emotionally engaged fashion, whereas the liveliest and most thoughtful group included those with high exhaustion scores. The paradox is understandable only if we accept that truly emotionally engaged practice *is* exhausting. This is not the same thing as burn out, but it can lead in that direction if individuals and teams have insufficient opportunity to process the emotional complexity of their experience so that they are capable of *staying* engaged and enduring the hardships of the work without the need to cut off and become unreceptive. Arguably, the crisis of staff recruitment and retention which afflicts so many health and social care settings these days may significantly be attributed to the absence of the right kind of supervisory and consultative support in teams and workplaces. If practice supervision in the end confers all the benefits upon staff which I am suggesting it does, we might ask why it is not embedded in a more widespread fashion in our structures of service delivery. Once again I think the answer lies partly in the double-edged nature of the experience of being fully engaged with the practice task. If the purpose of the supervisory space is to create a context for sustained thinking about emotional experience and dynamics, including most importantly the painful dimensions of this experience, it is hardly surprising to find a trend working against the introduction and maintenance of supervisory spaces. Everyone is inclined not to want to think about painful matters, and healthcare professionals, including those specialising in mental health, are no exception. Resistance to the introduction of regular supervision in agencies is therefore common, just as individuals may resist or be deeply ambivalent about the opportunity that supervision provides. This basic dynamic is one to which supervisors must always be alert, and which, at the organisational level, managers and leaders may have to struggle with over some period of time in search of a change of culture in their agency with respect to supervision. Under the best of circumstances, trust in supervision can break down if the forces acting on a particular worker or team are too painful or overwhelming. The following story is taken from my own experience as a practitioner in a community social work team nearly 20 years ago. But its themes are as applicable today as they were then.

A painful incident

In this generic social work team I specialised in mental health social work and was a mental welfare officer with powers under the Mental Health Act. I had a client, a young man with a diagnosis of paranoid schizophrenia who at the time was trying to live independently in his own flat, which I had helped him obtain. However, he had suffered a deterioration in his condition and had accepted voluntary admission to the local, community-based psychiatric hospital. His state of mind, and some of his behaviour, had led me and others in his professional and personal network to become extremely concerned about him so I called a meeting of the main professionals involved, including his psychiatrist, to try and assess how best to respond, taking account of the various risks he seemed to pose to himself at the time. After much deliberation it was decided that there was nothing to be gained from detaining him compulsorily, and that the present arrangements for support and management were adequate and well worked out. Two days later he walked out of hospital, went back to his flat and mutilated himself in a most dramatic, painful and disturbing manner.

At this time, as was normal then in local authority social work, I was supervised weekly for an hour or an hour and a half by my team leader. She was an experienced, exceptionally thoughtful, reflective, and enabling figure, with high professional standards and very committed to the professional development of her staff. Her ethos was that while time was precious, so, by and large, it was the responsibility of supervisees to contain their questions and anxieties and bring them in a prepared way to the weekly meeting; she was also flexible and readily available in emergency or extremity. I was deeply distressed by the incident, and felt profoundly and irrationally guilty. But I did not go to my supervisor. Three days later when I told her about events in our usual meeting, she looked at me in astonishment and said, 'Why on earth didn't you come to me before?' I think the answer had something to do with being myself in a state somewhat akin to trauma. Unable to think clearly about what had happened, I felt directly and almost causally responsible, as though without a doubt I should have acted to prevent this tragedy. My inability to avail myself of understanding, thought and of an opportunity to begin to process events and their emotional effect upon me was partly an act of self-condemnation in which I held that I must suffer, and suffer alone for what happened. Now, this is an entirely unproductive response, even if it is in some sense an understandable one. If perpetuated, it could only have led to a form of damage to my professional self-esteem and effective continued professional functioning. Such incidents do occur, and we must expect them to occur, and I propose that it is part of our professional responsibility towards ourselves, both individually and collectively, that we create, sustain and all importantly *make good use of* conditions under which we can process the variety of emotional effects arising from our practice.

Cultures of understanding, cultures of blame

We see here an environment in which supervisory understanding was well established in an agency, and in an important sense in my own mind. But, in the face of an intensely distressing experience, much more primitive feelings and reactions are mobilised. A culture of blame, persecution, shame and despair may set in very quickly in both the internal world of the practitioner and in the external world of formal accountability processes. These may quickly supplant more benign trends towards understanding and thought. If an organisational policy or political culture of fear and anxiety about admitting, or exploring, our part in tragedies and professional errors prevents us in any way from availing ourselves of an opportunity for thoughtful reflection and learning from experience, individually or collectively, this has serious implications for how we manage the all-important boundary between the requirement for professional scrutiny or self-scrutiny and the need for space in which to learn from experience and to repair damage to ourselves, which can arise from our participation in the work we do. We need an appropriately benign self-critical and self-examining capacity if we are to truly learn from experience; we need to be able to face up to our acts of negligence and error, to be capable of analysing them, understanding them and putting them to use in the service of professional self-improvement. And the fact is that the vast majority of ordinary professional doctors and healthcare professionals have this readily available to them. But the judgement of our times is that this dimension of our working lives, in which traditional forms of professional self-accountability arise from the internal professional systematisation of the ordinary human capacity for critical self-reflection, is inadequate to meet the demands of maintaining rigorous standards in public life. The problem is that externally driven methodologies for achieving such accountability threaten to tear the heart out of the meaning of what it is to be professional. This is the precarious environment in which the practice of reflective supervision is now located.

Defences: mental and physical

A couple of years after this painful incident occurred, a colleague of mine was assaulted in the reception area of the office by a woman who grabbed his testicles. Although he was not badly injured, the degree of intrusion, shock and shame was too much for the whole team to bear. A decision was quickly taken to introduce various physical security measures in the reception area – glass screens, security buzzers and so on. Possibly, these measures were justified in terms of reducing the likelihood of further incidents, but equally there is evidence that 'security' of this kind may contribute to a deterioration of relationships between a community and its health and welfare services, escalating rather than reducing the possibility of violence. However, staff will almost certainly feel safer, even if the objective risks stay much the same. The situation is analogous to one in which we 'cut off' and erect emotional barriers to protect us from the intrusion of the mental pain of other people. We may feel safer, but our capacity to do the work through the medium of relationships – which in the last analysis are all we really have – is damaged. The receptivity of an agency to its clientele is often writ large in the arrangements one encounters at the first point of contact, which is, literally and metaphorically, the 'reception' area. Supervision practices may or may not contribute to maintaining receptivity at the organisational as well as the personal level, but the *ethos* they embody is identical in each case.

Conflict and mirroring

Usually, feelings are not communicated by means of actual physical violence. But they are often passed on to us with a force that can feel like emotional violence or intrusion. In psychoanalytic thinking and practice, which I believe still provides us with the best way of understanding how people function emotionally, it is assumed that we never entirely outgrow the states of mind which were typical of our earliest life. Illness, bereavement, loss of all kinds or marital conflicts can serve to throw us back on our earliest ways of feeling and behaving, and we become incapable of managing or 'containing' our anxieties, furies, disappointments and resentments. We may not be aware that we are doing it, but most often we will then resort to ridding ourselves of these states into other people. Healthcare workers are frequently made the receptacles for their patients' unmanageable states of mind. As described above, this will probably leave us feeling bad, in turn, often without quite being able to identify how the bad feeling came about. But there are more subtle and complicated processes that occur when difficult feelings are being passed around, and supervisors often find they are part of the 'not so wonderful' chain of people who become involved. Below I describe an exchange which occurred in supervision with a very experienced practitioner who now has a role managing national educational and training developments.

> The practitioner came to me for regular sessions and I could detect that she was in a state of some agitation. She described a situation in which she and a group of colleagues who work in a rather dispersed organisational environment had gathered with their own senior management for a kind of 'Away Day' that was supposed to include an element of peer supervision. It seemed that someone had made a reference during the day to the senior management group using this event as a kind of expensive day's holiday from work. This comment, whatever it was, had got back to the Chief Executive who e-mailed the whole group later that night expressing her annoyance at the implications of the remark. The practitioner went on to describe quite separately how she felt compromised by an organisational decision emanating from her immediate manager that had left her to implement what she called a 'fudged' policy process which was already showing signs of rebounding rather seriously. Two days earlier she had received a difficult phone call from a regional manager threatening wholesale withdrawal from an important, expensive and well-established training initiative in consequence. The problem for me listening to the practitioner's account was that I found it incoherent, and I interrupted several times seeking clarification. I was aware of irritation building up in me each time I did this, and I was half-aware that this was probably communicating itself

to the practitioner, until the point came where I saw her eyes redden and she burst into tears. This is someone with whom I had had 18 months' constructive, and I think in her experience, productive and helpful supervision. So, it would seem that with even the best of intentions support can sometimes be rapidly transformed *into* persecution. How might we understand what is happening here?

I think the organising theme of the material brought by the practitioner was conflict, conflict experienced as persecutory and disabling rather than as an emotional experience that could be named and processed. Whatever had or had not been voiced by one of her peers in relation to their management, it seemed to have been experienced as hostile and attacking, resulting in a response from the Chief Executive which was felt, in turn, to be retaliatory and critical. Further, the practitioner experienced herself as being landed with the task of defending a contradictory organisational position, for which she was being held responsible. My impression was that the practitioner felt herself to be powerless in the face of a difficulty within her own organisation in clearly facing up to a possibly painful policy decision. The effect was to render her internally conflicted, and angry, but not quite able at the point she brought the material to me to think straight about the whole situation. Her uncharacteristic incoherence when she presented her work in supervision with me seemed to mask a good deal of anger which was somehow 'projected' into me. I, in turn, failed to process this adequately, and my rather snappy responses *led to an exact mirroring or replication of the supervisee's own experience of her relationship to her own management.* A complex and conflicted state of affairs is brought to supervision, but is first of all *enacted between* us rather than made available for reflective thought. The conflict is seemingly too much to think about for a whole sequence of people, including myself at first. So it keeps being passed on until someone succeeds in responding differently. After the practitioner burst into tears, I felt compassionate about her situation and rather guilty about my response. I was able to say something more empathic to her about what seemed to be her internally conflicted state and sense of powerlessness. This seemed to help her to articulate matters in a more lucid way, and I also said that I thought what really triggered her bursting into tears were my own rather irritable reactions. She agreed, and I said that something about the relationship between her and her senior managers seemed to have been played out between us here in the room.

From here it was possible to move on to do some further thinking about how the practitioner might be able to define the problem she has been left with as an 'organisational conflict', which she could take back to her managers and ask them to reconsider from within their organisational roles rather than as a 'hot potato' being passed between managers and the participant in an ultimately futile manner. So, through thinking, or the capacity for thought, in such situations we can discover how to be *in charge* of rather than *unknowingly driven* by the complex and powerful feelings that inevitably attend the kind of work we do. We are all under pressure to know how to act in such circumstances, but we are often pushed into action before we have had proper time and space to think. The capacity to think better under fire, although never perfectly achievable, seems to me to be a core aspiration for the kind of work we do. The development of this capacity may only really be achieved through skilled supervision, which most of us may go on needing for most of our professional lives, and there is nothing to be in the least ashamed of in this. Because the kinds of enactments I have described in the extract from my own experience are common, but are also vital sources of information about the hidden emotional dynamics driving a particular situation, supervision is itself a highly skilled process.

These kinds of enactments have been vividly explored by psychotherapists who went out and worked in front-line settings in order to experience for themselves the kinds of pressures that staff are under, whilst providing intensive supervision groups to the practitioners who they worked alongside. In their book, *Mate and Stalemate*, Janet Mattinson and Ian Sinclair (1979) make a classic study of the charged and difficult dynamics that often threaten to engulf workers but which, if thought about and understood, may be put to the service of helping patients and preserving more receptive organisations for patients and staff to relate to.

Conclusion

This chapter has not presented a 'model' or 'framework' for providing supervision. Other writers in this book have offered thoughts about these; the main aim here has been to emphasise the importance of the emotional receptivity of supervisors to the experience of supervisees, who in turn need to be emotionally available in their day-to-day work. The chapter assumes that the great majority of practitioners are 'competent' in the familiar sense of that word. But, in the face of acute or chronic mental pain, emotional deprivation, anxieties about illness or dying – indeed any of the infinite variety of distress encountered in primary care settings – all of us are frequently rendered emotionally and practically 'incompetent'. Supervisors are no more mature or immune to the effect of difficult states of mind than anyone else, but the thoughtfulness of the supervisory space is an essential bulwark against the harmful impact of the burden and confusion which patients and users may experience, and ask us to share. Not only are we entitled to this form of self-protection, but the understanding which accompanies it is vital to the task of enduring in the face of the difficulties of the work. In the end, supervision is not for the worker, but for the patient.

References

Daws D (1995) Consultation in general practice. In: J Trowell and M Bower (eds) *The Emotional Needs of Young Children and their Families: using psychoanalytic ideas in the community*. Routledge, London.

Mattinson J and Sinclair I (1979) *Mate and Stalemate*. Basil Blackwell, Oxford.

PART III

Practical approaches

CHAPTER 6

Nursing supervision in primary care

Sylvia Debreczeny

Introduction

Clinical supervision is now a recognised and accepted part of the process of personal and professional development in nursing practice, although some confusion remains about the process itself, the purpose of supervision (especially with regard to outcomes) and the models to be followed.

The United Kingdom Central Council for Nursing Midwifery and Health Visiting (UKCC) has provided guidance on this process and various writers have been influential in applying this to practice (for example, Butterworth and Faugier 1992; Morton-Cooper and Palmer 2000; Proctor 1989). Ghayle and Lillyman (2000) point out that the concept is not unfamiliar to nurses, including as it does elements of mentoring, facilitation and preceptorship, practices which have been used in conjunction with the Project 2000 pre-registration training programme since the late 1980s. However, the purpose of clinical supervision as a tool, and in particular as the preferred method of development, is relatively recent, and the emphasis on reflection, both in and on practice, links it to government initiatives for personal development planning, portfolios and clinical governance.

Wherever it is used, it is understood that clinical supervision is designed to be an educational and developmental system, rather than a managerial one, thus ensuring that ownership rests with the practitioner. Using an informal strategy of skilled and expert advice and discussion, supervisees should be encouraged to use the process to develop their skills, to seek supportive help from fellow professionals or to address the managerial and quality aspects of practice.

So why is this different in primary care? This may be considered from a number of angles, not least because of the relative recency of practice nursing as a career path, because of the professional isolation of many practice nurses and because of the employment relationship between the nurse and GPs. Any or all of these features may well preclude fruitful development through clinical supervision. However, by addressing these issues and devising appropriate models, this process may yet be included as a valuable learning system in this branch of the profession.

Clinical supervision as a preferred method of professional development

Clinical supervision is described by the UKCC (1996) as a method of support which enables nurses to develop their skills, knowledge and professional understanding throughout their career. This is defined in the *Position Statement* (UKCC 1996) in more practical terms as being:

> to identify solutions to problems, improve practice and increase understanding of professional issues.

Nursing has long been recognised as a profession which demands a heavy and continuous intellectual and emotional commitment from its practitioners, and this has become increasingly evident as professional accountability, extended roles and increased patient involvement have developed. The UKCC requires practitioners to commit to a form of post-registration education throughout their professional life, recommending five days of education every three years as a minimum standard for the development needed to meet these challenges.

However, changes in health practices and policies have required practitioners to provide evidence of ongoing development, which cannot be fully met by traditional forms of education, nor is this in fact desirable. Experienced professionals are more likely to be able to learn from their practice by considering their actions, identifying the gaps in their knowledge, seeking individual solutions to meet their needs and applying the new knowledge and skills to amend, update or modify their practice. This concept of reflective learning, classically described by Schon (1987), and by many others, as the 'learning cycle', is the model preferred by the UKCC (1996) which proclaimed that:

> Clinical supervision is a practice-focused professional relationship involving a practitioner reflecting on practice guided by a skilled supervisor.

It is now also recommended as the basis of the personal development planning needed for clinical governance, by the Department of Health, and in the Chief Medical Officer's report.

For nurses, this form of development is welcome and generally familiar, with the noted similarities to mentorship and preceptorship. Mentorship in nursing education is regarded as an informal nurturing relationship between an experienced professional and a novice, usually throughout training. Preceptorship is seen to be a rather more formal teaching relationship, particularly used for newly qualified nurses, but still enabling the more junior to learn from the experienced practitioner. Neither role is seen to be judgemental (for instance, as an assessor or examiner would be) but is used to guide and develop individuals in their professional role, to improve their practice skills and enhance their self-awareness and confidence. Clinical supervision is an extension of this practice and may be conducted between nurses of the same or different grades, expertise and clinical interest, or even between nurses and other health professionals.

However, while the idea is sound, difficulties in implementation may well be anticipated given the many different clinical environments in which nursing takes place and the varied nature of nursing practice. The UKCC recommendations (1996) attempt to anticipate difficulties by suggesting that no single format should be recommended, either for the process or for the choice of supervisors, stating instead that:

> the process ... should be developed by practitioners and managers according to local circumstances. Ground rules should be agreed so that practitioners and supervisors approach clinical supervision openly, confidently and are aware of what is involved.

A common consensus appears to be that whilst everyone should have access to clinical supervision, it may be necessary to adapt the process to suit both the clinical setting and the practitioners. There is also some agreement that supervision should follow a holistic approach and may be used to address clinical, professional, managerial and personal issues. It requires commitment from both supervisors and supervisees, to agree appropriate meeting times, set the ground rules, undertake necessary preparation and keep records of meetings. It may also involve both parties agreeing and signing a learning contract. Management support is also needed, and adopting clinical supervision as part of the overall development strategy for the organisation will demonstrate commitment and recognition of the value of this process.

The nature of practice nursing

This is a relative recent career option for nurses, dating from the introduction of the Family Doctors' Charter in 1966, when a system of financial reimbursement enabled GPs to employ nurses to provide a wider range of services. Prior to this, general practice was mainly concerned with responding to illness and district nurses provided any nursing services that might have been required. However, GPs gradually came to recognise the benefits of multiprofessional primary healthcare teams in promoting health rather than simply responding to illness. With the implementation of the 1990 contract for general practice, when a more proactive approach involving health promotion, surveillance and disease management was required, the role of the practice nurse has taken on a more professional focus.

Practice nurses now have an acknowledged career pathway, with opportunities for academic development and increased scope for practice. They are able to extend their role by taking responsibility for monitoring patients with chronic diseases, such as asthma or diabetes, providing health advice and sometimes prescribing. They also contribute to the development of practice protocols and may be involved in practice management.

However, despite this increased opportunity, practice nurses are difficult to recruit in many parts of the country. Many choose practice nursing for the flexibility it offers and work part-time hours in order to meet family commitments. Any one nurse could be the only nurse working in a practice with several GPs and have limited contact with other practice nurses, either in the practice or outside it. Their professional development might depend on the goodwill of their employing GP, relying on his awareness of the advantages of professional development. Anecdotal evidence suggests that the practice nurse will often undertake professional development in her own time and at her own expense, even when the outcome is directly applicable to practice. These conditions put practice nurses in a unique position, as nurses invariably work in teams, with a clear management structure and peer group support.

Clinical supervision is particularly appropriate in this field of nursing, with manifold opportunities for improving interprofessional working, patient relationships and clinical skills. However, the nature of the role does create some problems, not least in identifying an appropriate supervisor, ensuring protected time and implementing outcomes into practice.

Developing an understanding of an appropriate concept of clinical supervision

It is recognised that while the concept of clinical supervision may be familiar and welcomed as being associated with recognition of a professional and mature approach to learning, the term has created anxiety among some nurses. General nurses, in particular, associate the supervision aspect as being a device for control and discipline, more in tune with authority than autonomy (Butterworth *et al.* 2001). The concept of supervision finds more favour among nurses working in mental health, where it has long been integral to patient care through case discussion. Here it is seen as being supportive, developmental and valuable in promoting competence.

One way of enabling practice nurses to appreciate the benefits of clinical supervision would be through the construction of an appropriate conceptual model. A conceptual model is usually understood as being a diagrammatic representation of essential components (in this case for professional develop-ment), clarifying the relationships between each part and linking into practice. The model can illuminate the concepts, the stages of the clinical supervision process and can identify the areas of knowledge and sources of support.

A conceptual model may take different forms. For instance, it could be a dia-gram or map or, alternatively, it could be produced in chart form, linking knowledge to practice, or written as a list of personal goals. Whatever structure the individual model may take, it should contain common elements such as commitment, professional responsibility, support, learning goals and outcomes (Barrowman 2000).

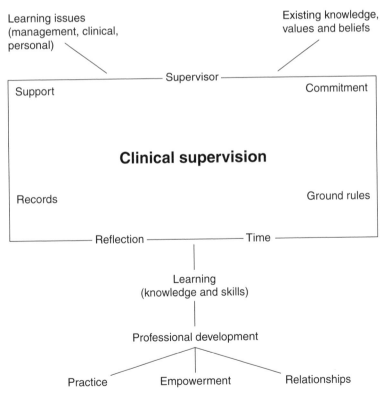

Figure 6.1   A conceptual model for clinical supervision.

As part of the preparation for clinical supervision, practice nurses could define the model of supervision most appropriate for them. This will not only encourage ownership of and commitment to learning but should also provide a practical focus by identifying the most appropriate areas for supervision in relation to their own practice, and ensuring that the goals of the supervisor and supervisee are congruent.

A personal model for clinical supervision is illustrated in Figure 6.1. Several needs might feed into the model of supervision. These could be the need for learning about specific matters, the need for clarification of value and beliefs, and the need to build on existing knowledge. Other factors might include the choice of supervisor, the commitment of both parties and agreed ground rules such as timing, confidentiality and non-judgemental attitudes. The projected outcomes of being supervised might include improvements in practice, increased personal empowerment and enhanced professional relationships.

The construction of such a conceptual framework also depends on how the main purpose of supervision is defined. Proctor (1991) suggested that it may be used for one of three purposes, which she describes as formative, normative or supportive. Formative supervision is concerned with developing skills and proficiency in practice, normative is linked to quality issues and the professional role, whereas restorative involves providing support and raising self-esteem.

The clarification of understanding of the main features, purposes and projective outcomes in this way enables individuals to concentrate on those aspects of development most pertinent to them. This makes the process of supervision and the way it is implemented personal and acceptable to individuals.

Setting up a supervision system for practice nurses

As may be seen from the above, setting up a system of supervision for practice nurses must take into account the variations in their working conditions. It is likely that individual circumstances, such as working single-handedly or for part-time hours, could well preclude the use of one specific formula, and a loose framework which may be tailored to the individual circumstances is likely to be more suitable.

Models for implementing clinical supervision depend on the type of working environment. Where supervision has been organised so that it reflects the commonality of experience (either in a large hospital department, with many staff doing the same job, or with a group of practice nurses) the success of the model is based, in part, on getting the structures right. A structure would be, for example, a supervision group.

Where nurses work in less homogeneous circumstances, such a highly organised and structured approach cannot be introduced with ease. An alternative system may have to be used, which concentrates more on the here and now possibilities for supervision, with supervision coming from someone immediately at hand (perhaps a working colleague). Such an approach is often poorly structured, but may be suited to addressing current problems. I call this approach a 'process approach' as it concentrates almost wholly on the process of one individual's working world.

Both these models could apply to practice nursing. A structured model could apply to larger practices, employing three or four nurses, who could set up a supervision group among themselves. Alternatively single-handed nurses could join a practice nurse forum or self-directed learning group for group supervision. An example of a process model could occur in a small practice, where the GP or a district nurse becomes the clinical supervisor to the practice nurse.

Either of these models could work perfectly well, but some potential difficulties immediately spring to mind. First, a group of colleagues working together may form a mutual support group rather than clinical supervision group, and could be too closely involved or cosy, hesitating to offer criticisms that could disrupt the relationship or lead to distress, however objectively offered.

The process model could also embody some of these difficulties, but even more crucial could be the nature of the supervisory relationship if one person is the employer and the other an employee, as could occur if the GP is the clinical supervisor to the practice nurse. It would not be surprising if the employee was reluctant to identify any problem that might indicate less than adequate competence, or to raise possible questions about her employer's behaviour.

With either approach, problems of confidentiality could arise. A lack of experience or training among supervisors could result in a failure to recognise learning needs or opportunities, leading to a situation of 'the blind leading the blind'.

It might be necessary for a practice nurse to seek more than one source of clinical supervision, depending on the purpose of supervision or the nature of the learning need. For instance, the practice nurse could raise issues of quality with her GP or a primary care tutor, discuss the acquisition of particular skills with a senior practice nurse or district nurse, and seek professional support from a peer group.

Whatever the format, some ground rules should be followed. For example, the purpose of supervision should be agreed, appropriate time set aside, relevant preparation undertaken and confidentiality assured.

Using supervision in practice

In order to illustrate how clinical supervision might work for a practice nurse, the following case studies demonstrate the different systems described above. All personal details have been altered.

Case study 1

Nurse G, a mature lady, has recently started working part time in a single-handed practice. Among her regular duties she notes that she will be required to carry out ear syringing when necessary. As this is a procedure she has not performed since her student days, she expresses her anxiety to her employer Dr X, who assures her that she will be fine as the process has not changed for years!

Nurse G has joined a supervision group consisting of seven other practice nurses that meets monthly and is supervised by a primary care development manager. She asks her colleagues for their opinion. The group asks questions: 'What previous experience has she had?' 'Who had carried out this process for Dr X before she started working in the practice?' 'How had she responded to Dr X's assurance?' This period of question and answer continues until the situation is clarified.

The supervisor then suggests that the group identifies the elements of this specific problem, for example personal lack of clinical skill, clinical credibility, professional accountability and the nature of her relationship with her employer.

The group discusses each aspect, with some members linking this situation to their own experience, and in doing so brainstorms some possible actions, for example observing the procedure by sitting in with another group member; identifying possible practice update courses to cover this and other procedures; meeting with Dr X and discussing Nurse G's professional role and accountability, etc.

Nurse G notes the comments for her portfolio, and plans how to follow up her need for professional development.

Case study 2

Nurse J is a single-handed practice nurse working full time in a group practice with four GPs. She has been running an asthma clinic fortnightly for the past six months, but patient attendance has been sporadic, despite her following the practice recall procedure. Nurse J wonders whether this is the most effective way for her to manage the asthma patients.

Nurse J does not have a regular clinical supervisor, usually seeking advice informally from what seems to be the most appropriate source. In this instance she decides to discuss this problem with one of her GP colleagues, Dr B, and arranges an appropriate time for a meeting, explaining to him what she would like to discuss.

Nurse J prepares for the meeting by collecting clinic attendance records, data from the asthma chronic disease register and details of the recall procedure. She phones several of her friends who are also practice nurses, to find out what they do. Dr B also prepares for the meeting by doing a quick literature search on the internet, and obtains information on alternative systems of monitoring patients.

At the meeting, Nurse J explains her problem with the clinic attendance and identifies some of the other issues, for example time management, administration and secretarial support, possible potential for updating in asthma care. Dr B asks a number of questions to clarify his understanding of the issues, explores Nurse J's relationship with the administrative staff in relation to the way that patients are recalled, and the extent of her computer skills in accessing records.

They discuss the value of the present system, the nursing time spent in organising the clinic and consider the alternative strategies. A preferred option is selected and they decide to confer with the practice team about introducing this. Nurse J also identified a number of personal learning needs, including managing change, teamwork and computer skills, and considered how to meet these. She recorded a note of the issues discussed and the outcomes of the meeting, for her personal portfolio.

Case study 3
Nurse A has been working three days a week as a practice nurse for the past two years. She works with two other part-time nurses in a busy group practice and, although she enjoys her work, does not really feel that she is progressing anywhere in her career. She has considered enrolling on a course or something similar, but with a lively three-year-old daughter and other family responsibilities, she is reluctant to make any long-term commitments.

Nurse A and her colleagues have arranged monthly clinical supervision sessions with a nurse practitioner (Nurse P) who works in neighbouring practice. However, Nurse A feels that she would prefer to discuss this issue in private, so arranges a separate meeting in her lunch break. Her supervisor suggests that she prepare for the meeting by completing a personal profile and self-appraisal form, identifying her strengths and weaknesses and goals for the next five years.

At the meeting, Nurse A begins by describing her situation, her feelings of frustration and her current problems. Nurse P invites her to expand on the nature of her commitments and they consider the effect of these on her work and professional development. Nurse P also enquires generally about Nurse A's health and whether she feels she is coping. Having been reassured about this, the discussion moves on to consider her working relationship with her colleagues and her responsibilities to the practice. A review of her personal profile and self-appraisal leads them to consider whether she is currently working to her strengths, and how these could be expanded. They are able to identify some areas of practice that Nurse A would like to develop and consider how to achieve this, given her present limitations.

Nurse A is invited to expand on her long-term goals and to suggest whether she can take any appropriate initial steps toward these. Lastly, they summarise the points discussed and agree to meet again in two months' time. Nurse A keeps a record of the meeting for her portfolio.

Evaluating the effects of clinical supervision

It is widely regarded that, for nurses, clinical supervision is the most appropriate way forward for professional development and improving patient care, but there appears to be little evidence of evaluation to support this.

So far, the evidence to support the effectiveness of this process has come from small-scale surveys or anecdotal evidence from practitioners, but the general consensus appears to be that the supervision process does produce a number of benefits, including reducing stress, improving morale and strengthening working relationships (Barrowman 2000; Butterworth *et al.* 2001). Unfortunately, it does not seem that any evaluation of the effect of clinical supervision on patient care has yet been undertaken, nor is it clear how this could be measured.

However, it may be argued that if the practice nurse is more confident and capable in the work setting, professional practice is likely to be improved and patients will benefit as a result. Management theorists such as Drucker (1994) support this argument, claiming that: 'People determine the performance capacity of an organisation'.

The key to that improvement seems to be the development of self-awareness through reflection, which, when applied to patient care, enables nurses to review their actions, to identify problems and to think through solutions. Skill in reflection is suggested as a hallmark of the expert practitioner, who works intuitively, solves problems in practice and develops new knowledge (Benner 1984).

Furthermore, a programme of ongoing development represented by a system of clinical supervision contributes to the creation of the learning organisation, in which the improvement in performance of individual practitioners is seen as making a significant difference to the quality of the output of the organisation (Sissons and Storey 2000).

Conclusion

The personal and professional demands of nursing in present times put a heavy responsibility on the individual for constant updating and improvement. Being aware of one's learning needs, whether clinical, theoretical or managerial, is an essential component of professional practice, and the chosen vehicle for maintaining this skill is clinical supervision.

Nurses have generally welcomed this form of professional development as it empowers individuals and enables them to develop their own systems of learning in support of practice. As nurses mostly work in clinical teams, the process is easily implemented and maintained. However, practice nurses may be the exception to this situation as they may be isolated from their peers by the nature of their work or their personal responsibilities.

Despite this, it is possible to devise a suitable and flexible system to accommodate their special circumstances and enable them to meet professional requirements for development through clinical supervision.

References

Barrowman LM (2000) *Clinical Supervision: the future imperatives*. NBNI Occasional Paper.

Benner P (1984) *From Novice to Expert: excellence and power in clinical nursing practice*. Addison Wesley, California.

Butterworth T and Faugier J (1992) *Clinical Supervision and Mentorship in Nursing*. Chapman & Hall, London.

Butterworth T, Faugier J and Burnard P (2001) *Clinical Supervision and Mentorship in Nursing*. Nelson Thornes, London.

Drucker PF (1994) *Managing the Non-Profit Organisation*. Butterworth–Heinemann, Oxford.

Ghayle T and Lillyman S (2000) *Effective Clinical Supervision*. Quay Books, Salisbury.

Morton-Cooper A and Palmer A (2000) *Mentoring, Preceptorship and Clinical Supervision*. Blackwell Science, Oxford.

Proctor B (1989) On being a trainer: training and supervision for counselling in action. In: P Hawkins and R Shohet (eds) *Supervision in the Helping Professions*. Open University Press, Milton Keynes.

Schon DA (1987) *Educating the Reflective Practitioner*. Basic Books, New York.

Sissons K and Storey J (2000) *The Realities of Human Resource Management*. Open University Press, Milton Keynes.

UKCC (1996) *Position Statement on Clinical Supervision for Nursing and Health Visiting*. UKCC, London.

CHAPTER 7

Balint groups and the Balint method

John Salinsky

History

The Balint group is probably one of the earliest methods of clinical supervision to be provided for family doctors. The group and the method are named after Michael Balint, a psychoanalyst originally from Hungary. He and his wife, Enid Balint, started a series of seminars in London in the 1950s with the aim of helping GPs to reach a better understanding of what they called 'the psychological aspect' of general practice. The method consisted of case presentation followed by general discussion, with the emphasis on the emotional content of the doctor–patient relationships. The seminar leaders were originally always psychoanalysts: nowadays a group may be led by a GP, a mental health professional or one of each. Whatever their professional background, all leaders need training and experience in the specific Balint method.

Although Michael and Enid Balint were psychoanalysts their aim was not to turn GPs into psychotherapists, but to help them to become more psychologically aware. Learning to listen with close attention to what a patient was saying was one of the most important skills which the early Balint group members were able to acquire – in a period when the teaching of what we now call 'communication skills' was unknown. Michael Balint's book, *The Doctor, his Patient and the Illness* (Balint 2000), became a key text in the renaissance of British general practice in the 1960s and the Balints' ideas achieved world-wide recognition. However, relatively few doctors ever took part in Balint groups in the UK and they were regarded with scepticism by the majority of GPs. In continental Europe (where talking about feelings is perhaps more acceptable) Balint groups have been considerably more widespread.

Groups for established doctors

The original Balint group members were doctors who had already been established in practice for several years. Many were becoming aware of the importance of psychological and psychosomatic problems among their patients and were feeling frustrated at their lack of ability to help. Their interest and their neediness provided the motivation necessary to attend a 90-minute group once a week for several years. Nowadays, because of increased time pressures, there are very few such groups and an interested GP principal may have to be content with an annual weekend Balint group. But, whatever the frequency, the established doctor will have plenty of problem patients to present. He may already have realised that some patients disturb him emotionally or provoke a withdrawal of empathy which impoverishes the relationship and reduces effectiveness. These 'traditional' Balint groups are easy to lead because everyone understands the aims of the group and it is easier to concentrate on the doctor–patient relationship without being distracted by other anxieties.

However, with a little modification, the Balint group can also be a very good way of supervising doctors in training. Michael Balint ran some groups for students in the 1960s and in Germany participation in a Balint group is part of the official medical student curriculum (Otten 1998). In the UK today, the chief beneficiaries of the Balint group are GP registrars whose course organisers, like myself, have some experience and training in the method. Here is a description of the GP registrar Balint group in action.

The Balint method and the GP registrar

GP registrars do not choose to join a Balint group – those on my course and a few others in the UK simply find that the group session forms part of the curriculum. Most of them welcome the opportunity to talk about their own work with patients and, after a while, they begin to realise that the interpersonal and emotional aspects of the consultation are among the chief difficulties that they are experiencing in the transfer from hospital to general practice.

The setting: structure of the groups

Balint sessions take place in the Postgraduate Centre in the second half of our weekly half-day release course. Because we have a total attendance of about 15 GP registrars and one or two GP senior house officers (SHOs) we divide into two groups for the Balint session. I lead one group and my course organiser colleague leads the other. Membership in each group remains fixed as far as possible so that group members can get used to working together and get to know each other better. Most registrars are with us for only a year, but some members of the three-year scheme manage to attend as SHOs at least on some occasions and are thus members of a group for three years. In many ways it is better to have two leaders so that they can complement each other and share the responsibility; however, we feel that it is more important for the groups not to become too big as this may make it difficult for people to talk freely about their work and themselves.

Ground rules

At the beginning of a year, we give a brief explanation of the purpose and aims of the group. We usually say that it will be an opportunity for the registrars to present and discuss patients who are of particular concern. These may be difficult or puzzling patients, or those who make the doctor feel uncomfortable. We are also interested in patients the doctor likes and is worried about but is not sure how to help. We say that the focus of discussion will be on what is happening in the doctor–patient relationship. We say that, in our experience, understanding the patient as a person is much the most difficult part of general practice. Registrars may not agree with this, especially in the early stages when they are more anxious about missing a physical diagnosis. We say that we are less concerned with finding solutions (though these will certainly be discussed) than with exploring and understanding what is going on. This should be acceptable as a restatement of advice always to reach a diagnosis before treatment. We are very interested in follow-up reports because hearing what happened in the next consultation is an excellent way of finding out whether the previous discussion was helpful to the presenting doctor.

Lastly, we suggest a few ground rules:

- everything said in the group will be treated as confidential, whether it is about patients, colleagues or group members themselves
- everyone should be heard and everyone's contribution should be respected
- although people can talk about their personal history if it seems relevant, there will be no unwelcome and intrusive questioning of group members about their own childhood experiences or losses.

Responsibilities of the group leader

The leader has to make sure that the ground rules, once agreed, are respected. He is responsible for starting and finishing the session on time. The available time is usually one hour and this usually accommodates two presentations.

One of these may be a follow-up from a previous discussion. During the session the leader needs to monitor how everyone in the group seems to be getting on. He may catch sight of someone trying unsuccessfully to get a word in – and will make a space for this individual. Alternatively, someone else may be talking too much and may need to be gently reminded that, although it is good to talk, it is also good to listen. As with any kind of small group work, it is vital for the members to feel that the group is a safe place in which to talk about how they feel, and how they have performed, without being criticised or ridiculed.

The work of the group

I will try to give an idea of what happens in one of my Balint group sessions and of my observations and interventions as group leader. This will be followed by an example of a typical case we have discussed.

The presentation

When everyone is settled I ask: '*Who has a patient they would like to talk about?*' I also remind the group that we are interested in follow-up consultations. There may be a long pause before someone speaks. In the early stages, people are nervous about presenting their work. I do not nominate anyone to bring a case the next week, so the presentations are spontaneous and delivered without notes. If there is more than one offer, we decide by mutual agreement who will go first. 'Urgent', that is, very distressing cases have priority.

The first presenting doctor then tells us about a patient. Doctors are allowed to speak without interruption until they have finished. I try to listen with as much concentration and encouragement as possible, and hope that this will provide a model of 'how to listen' for everyone else, should they need it.

During the presentation I observe the mood, the tone of voice and the body language of the narrator to get an idea of how talking about the patient is affecting the doctor emotionally. Some presentations are delivered in a low voice with downcast eyes; others are full of animation and include direct quotation of the patient's words or gestures. Some express the doctor's anxiety and feeling of helplessness. All these emotions are easily caught by the group members who begin to experience them too.

What kind of stories do we hear in these presentations? Typical problems include:

- the patient with chronic, medically unexplained symptoms or psycho-somatic symptoms

- patients who make what seem to be inappropriate demands for prescriptions, certificates, letters and referrals to specialists or for expensive investigations such as MRI scans
- patients who are rude or sarcastic, especially those who point out the registrar's extreme youth and lack of experience
- patients who make the doctor feel confused
- family conflicts: adolescent and marital problems
- difficulties in understanding someone from another culture
- worryingly depressed patients who hint at suicide
- patients who just might have a serious physical disorder in spite of their bad behaviour.

The phase of enquiry

When the presenting doctor has finished, he or she is thanked and I ask if anyone has any questions about matters of fact in the narrative which might have been missing or gone unheard. Such questions might be: 'How old is the patient?' 'What does he look like?' 'Does she have a partner?' I explain that a Balint group works better if presenters are spared questions at this stage about their own feelings with regard to patients or why they did certain things – or what they intend to do next. I want to avoid a situation in which the presenter is being bombarded with questions of this kind. This may seem strange to those who are more used to a different style of supervision, but there is a reason for it. Too much questioning of the presenter prevents the other group members from exploring and reflecting on their own thoughts about the story they have heard and the feelings it has induced in them. They need to wonder, to themselves and out loud, how the patient is feeling, what he or she really wants from the doctor, how they would feel if they were in the doctor's shoes.

The 'push back' phase

In order to avoid interrogation of the presenter I will often ask for an end to questions after a few minutes or when they cease to be purely factual. I will then ask presenters to move their chair back a few symbolic inches and then, whilst continuing to listen, to take no further active part in the discussion for about 20 minutes. This is called the 'push back' phase. During this time group members are asked not to direct questions or statements specifically to the presenter. The group members soon get the idea of this game and are usually happy to go along with it. They are now free to get to work on the case themselves using their experience, their imagination and, most importantly, their own emotional reactions. After an appropriate time (usually about 20 minutes) presenters are invited to rejoin the group and share their thoughts.

To begin with, the discussion is often quite medical. The group may try to reach a physical or psychiatric diagnosis. They may suggest referral to a consultant or to a counsellor or social worker. If the patient is making worrying demands on the doctor the group may try to protect him or her by recommending strict limits on prescribing, issuing of certificates or frequency of consultation. There may be a tendency to generalise away from the presented patient to the difficulties which GP registrars have in common: such as insufficient time, pressure to see too many patients, inexperience or vulnerability. Group members may introduce similar patients of their own so that the original patient is abandoned. In this situation, as group leader, I have to decide how long to let the discussion go on in this way before intervening. I want to let everyone have their say and express their concerns. But I also need, sooner or later, to bring the focus back to 'the patient as a person' and the emotional interaction between one doctor and one patient. Otherwise, although the discussion may be fruitful, the specific benefits of the Balint process will be lost.

The group leader's interventions

If the group is concentrating on the doctor–patient relationship the leader may need to do very little. He monitors the discussion and, if he feels that it is drifting off course, he applies a gentle touch to the tiller in order to bring it back. Interventions are often in the form of open questions, addressed to the group as a whole rather than to individuals. The question can be turned into a statement, such as: '*I wonder how the patient was feeling at the end of that consultation . . .*'

The leader might also ask (or wonder) how group members are feeling about the patient: do they like the individual, feel sorry for, feel angry with or feel indifferent towards them? What does the patient want from this doctor? What sort of doctor does the patient want the presenter to be? It is customary to avoid technical terms such as 'projection' or 'transference'. But the aim is to encourage the group members to be aware of their own feelings and to experience some empathy. This may not be easy to begin with as the group members need to feel safe enough to lower the defences which have so far protected them from 'emotional involvement' with their patients. And, indeed, sharing and feeling some of the pain of a distressed patient can be quite bruising.

If the emotional engagement with a single patient is too uncomfortable, the discussion may tend to head for calmer waters. The presenter may be reassured by a generalisation ('patients with a personality disorder are untreatable; there is nothing you can do'). Presenters may be advised to refer patients to a specialist agency and to minimise their own involvement. The leader might then intervene to say that specialist advice would indeed be helpful, but the patient will continue to need a GP and the role of the group is to try to understand what is going on in the current doctor–patient relationship.

If the group is really in danger of forgetting the existence of the presented patient, the leader may bring patients back into the discussion by representing them; he might say: '*If I were that patient I would be feeling very lost and abandoned: I would feel there was nobody to take care of me . . .*' This sort of intervention can be quite a powerful reviver of the group's willingness to experience feelings.

In general, leader interventions have the aim of encouraging the group members to stay with their feelings and to risk a little empathy with the patient. The leader will invite speculation about and reflection on patients' relationships and their inner world. He will try to help them, by example, to tolerate uncertainty, ambiguity and periods of silence.

How does a Balint session end?

Because we are not seeking solutions, the end is often inconclusive. The leader will not, as a rule, summarise the discussion or make any statement about what has been achieved. He will not make any recommendations for further management of this or any similar case. He will usually thank presenters for providing a case and ask them to give a follow-up report when they feel ready to do so.

Case study

Presentation
Lucy (a GP registrar) presented a young woman of 27 (Yvette) whose records showed she was always turning up 'inappropriately' at Saturday morning surgeries. The patient had an extensive skin rash whose management was difficult. Her usual GP was waiting for advice from the hospital clinic about a change of treatment, but the patient had failed her latest appointment. The patient was quite reluctant to reveal the full extent of her rash. Lucy did her best to examine her and explained the situation. Then she decided she must educate her about not coming on Saturdays because there was not enough time in a five-minute emergency slot to deal with her complicated problem. Yvette said: '*You doctors are all the same*' and called Lucy '*a discompassionate bitch*'. Lucy was shocked and hurt but did not retaliate. She continued the consultation and spent about half an hour with the patient altogether. She tried to explain that a weekday consultation would be more helpful, but everything she said to Yvette went '*in one ear and out of the other*'. Lucy asked Yvette when she left to make a double appointment on a weekday in five weeks' time: but she didn't. Lucy finished by asking how other people would deal with the problem.

Discussion

After expressing sympathy for Lucy's bad experience, the group immediately moved to the general problem of how to educate or discipline patients with ongoing problems that needed regular review not to come on Saturdays.

I let this go on until my discomfort was too great. I wanted to get the group back on the Balint track of looking at the individual doctor–patient relationship.

I reminded the group that this was the main purpose of the group and said I thought that we might learn more about the general problem also if we tried to understand Lucy's patient, Yvette, better. Why did they think she had behaved in this outrageous way? What sort of person was she? Lucy said Yvette worked in the City as a personal assistant. Someone said that she probably had a very stressful job and was treated very badly and 'discompassionately' at work. Other people said that Yvette was completely self-centred and did not care a damn about other people's feelings. She wanted to make Lucy feel bad and she had succeeded. Someone asked if she had a relationship and when Lucy said she was single, people smiled and said they were not surprised. Lucy said that Yvette had behaved like a child and someone else said it was like a tantrum. There was some brief speculation about whether she had had an unhappy childhood.

I asked how people thought Yvette had felt on leaving the surgery. Someone said she might have felt some remorse but others thought this was unlikely. The dread phrase 'personality disorder' was mentioned. There was general agreement that Yvette was a very unhappy person, ashamed and humiliated about her unsightly skin. Perhaps she was jealous of Lucy who was clearly a successful professional woman of about the same age with no skin problems.

I asked if the fact that Yvette was unhappy made the group feel any more liking and concern for her. There was cautious endorsement of this idea. But how can you help someone who is so negative and deliberately messes things up?

I asked: '*What sort of help does she really need; what would you do if she was your sister?*' One of the women said: '*Give her a good slap on the face!*' After some laughter, there were more serious comments about her needing some love and attention but it would be very difficult to provide because she seemed to relieve her feelings by trying to hurt or annoy people. Lucy remembered that, as she left, Yvette gave her a cheeky grimace as if to say '*So there!*' After this I said little because the group seemed to be more focused, concentrating on the relationship and not being side-tracked. At the end Lucy said she would be quite prepared to see the patient again and was not frightened of her. She promised to provide a follow-up if there was another consultation.

How might the Balint group help? Objectives and hopes

As a result of regular participation in a series of Balint groups, I would hope that the GP registrars would:

- feel listened to, supported and understood when they present cases
- become more tolerant of 'difficult' patients
- be more empathic to patients' feelings, including negative ones
- become more aware of their own feelings in the consultation and be able to use them in reaching a diagnosis
- allow their natural curiosity about patients as people to emerge
- gain some insight into why they find some patients particularly difficult or disturbing.

How far are these expectations realised? I asked the registrars to give me their impressions of how they experienced the Balint sessions and audio-recorded the discussion for about 20 minutes. This is a summary of the themes that emerged, with some quotations to illustrate them.

- **Overcoming isolation:** '*It's good to get other people's opinions . . . how they would deal with it.*' '*After hospital, you feel very isolated in general practice.*' '*No one else sees the patient. It's scary. Good to talk with your peer group.*' '*Everyone feels exactly the same – it's a real confidence builder.*'
- **Clinical uncertainty:** '*My first worry was, how do I cope clinically.*' '*How many people will die because I've missed the diagnosis?*'
- **Doctor–patient relationship:** '*Realised how important it is.*' '*What do people come for?*' '*Not just about clinical problems.*' '*We need to know more about how they developed.*' '*Important to keep an open mind.*'
- **Group leader's role:** '*You want to steer us away from the medical side towards the psychological. To look at what's behind . . .*'
- **See patient as a human being:** '*I am much more patient-centred now. The group helped me with that.*' '*It reminds you what general practice is all about.*' '*Hospital medicine is all about "they–they–they". We try to remember there is a human being sitting there. Not coming to attack you, coming for help. I feel more sympathetic*

towards them. It seems muddled but there's always a good reason why the patient has come.'

- **Dealing with fears of being thought inadequate:** *'Do they know who we [GP registrars] are?' 'They just know we are young.' 'Often they really wanted to see one of the partners, the doctor they know.'*

Does Balint have a lasting effect in creating 'a culture of supervision'?

Doctors who have taken part in Balint groups may be divided into:

- those who had a brief exposure, did not much like it and have no further use for it
- those who were in a group for a year or more, never returned to it, but still regard it as a positive experience
- those who continued to be interested, joined a Balint Society (in the UK or elsewhere) and continued to participate in groups when possible throughout their careers, either as members or group leaders or both.

Sadly, there is no satisfactory quantitative data on the first two groups. Those in the first category may have been in an inadequately led group or may simply have been temperamentally unsuited to this form of supervision. The evidence about the second group is so far only anecdotal. Nevertheless, leading members of the profession have publicly acknowledged the lasting benefits of their youthful experience in a Balint group (Horder 2001; Southgate 2000).

The third group, the Balint Society members, self-evidently continue to see Balint work as an important part of continuing professional development. There are at present few opportunities in the UK for established doctors to join ongoing groups. Enthusiasts have to be content with weekend groups, such as The Balint Society's annual Oxford meeting. In France and Belgium, Balint groups are much more widespread and in Germany, where the Balint Society has more than 1000 members, the method has become a recognised part of the curriculum of training and supervision for students, trainee family doctors (and psychiatrists) and mature GPs.

Research on the effectiveness of Balint groups

In the last few years we have seen the beginnings of a serious attempt to evaluate the effectiveness of Balint groups by looking for evidence of a change in attitudes and values in those who have experienced the process. Work is also being conducted on comparing the development of groups of doctors who have experienced Balint training with those who have not. The early stages of some of these projects were described in the International Balint Congresses in Oxford, England (Ludwig-Becker 1998), and Portoroz, Slovenia. Both quantitative and qualitative methods are being used. Preliminary results suggest that young family doctors who are Balint-trained are more psychologically skilled (Turner and Margo 1998), more tolerant of patients whose diagnosis is uncertain, more reflective and more aware of their own feelings about patients (Ludwig-Becker 1998). They have a greater degree of job satisfaction, are more able to tolerate feelings of helplessness and are less likely to suffer from burn out (Mandel *et al.* 2001). They have a more holistic approach, a more positive attitude to psychosomatic disorders, greater work satisfaction and are less likely to refer patients or order unnecessary tests (Kjeldmand 1998). In the next few years, these and other projects are likely to develop further and achieve publication.

Conclusions

Taking part in a Balint group involves time and commitment. Unless a suitable number of doctors in a locality can be found (ideally 8–10) the group will not be viable. A suitably trained and experienced leader or leaders will need to be available and everyone will need to commit to a regular meeting over a period of at least a year. Course organisers who wish to run Balint groups for GP registrars have the advantage of a ready-made group, but they may feel insufficiently skilled to act as Balint group leaders. Given these difficulties does the Balint group offer anything that makes the effort to start one worthwhile?

Other forms of supervision for GPs may provide excellent evaluation and mentoring of doctors' clinical skills, diagnostic reasoning and ability to evaluate evidence. But the important emotional component of medicine (Mandel *et al.* 2001), which can be painful to examine, may be avoided and glossed over. The Balint group is a unique supervision method whose chief concern is with the sensitivity of the doctor to the emotions of both doctor and patient. Greater awareness will lead to better understanding and enable doctors to mobilise their emotional intelligence in the interests of both their patients and themselves.

References

Balint M (2000) *The Doctor, his Patient and the Illness*. Churchill Livingstone, Edinburgh.

Horder J (2001) The first Balint group. *Br J Gen Prac*. **51**: 1038–39.

Kjeldmand D (1998) Has Balint activity by general practitioners any effect? In: J Salinsky (ed.) *Proceedings of the 11th International Balint Congress*. Limited Edition Press, Southport.

Ludwig-Becker (1998) Implementing Balint's method within the clinical department of a medical college. In: J Salinsky (ed.) *Proceedings of the 11th International Balint Congress.* Limited Edition Press, Southport.

Mandel A, Maoz B, Berger M and Narde Y (2001) An evaluation of Balint and Balint-like groups. In: *Abstracts from the 12th International Balint Congress.* (www.internationalbalintcongress.de/portorz/abstracts.htm)

Otten H (1998) Balint work in Germany. *Journal of the Balint Society.* **26**: 16–19.

Southgate L (2000) Foreword. In: J Salinsky and P Sackin *What Are You Feeling Doctor? Identifying and avoiding defensive patterns in the consultation.* Radcliffe Medical Press, Oxford.

Turner A and Margo G (1998) Overhead projections: the effect of Balint and non-Balint training on residents' skills and group comfort. In: J Salinsky (ed.) *Proceedings of the 11th International Balint Congress.* Limited Edition Press, Southport.

CHAPTER 8

A narrative-based approach to primary care supervision

John Launer

Background

In 1995 a group of us at the Tavistock Clinic in London began to teach a regular course for GPs and nurses from primary care. We came from a variety of backgrounds, including general practice, child psychiatry, clinical psychology and social work, but were all trained as family therapists as well. We hoped to use family therapy ideas to look at the whole range of primary care work – not just family work but also everyday consultations with individuals. We also wanted to use the ideas to look at the wider context of primary care, including practices, teams and the wider social and political systems surrounding these (Launer and Lindsey 1997).

One of our intentions was to provide an alternative to the more traditional 'Balint groups' for GPs that had originated at the Tavistock Clinic and have run there for nearly 50 years (Balint 1957; Gosling and Turquet 1964). Although we valued much that the Balint movement offered, including the importance placed on telling stories, we wanted to try something quite different. We aimed to offer skills training rather than case discussion alone. Instead of focusing mainly on the doctor–patient relationship, we wanted as well to encourage professionals from primary care to pay more attention to how people interact within their families, workplaces and in the other human systems that surround them. We also wanted to teach a course that was multidisciplinary.

Our courses have now been going for eight years, and in that time we have developed both our thinking and our approach to teaching in many ways. Most importantly, we think and teach far less these days about 'systems' like families and teams. We concentrate more on the stories, or 'narratives', that people tell. This is very much in keeping with changes in contemporary psychology and also within medicine – as discussed below.

Through our teaching we have also become aware that clinicians in primary care have an enormous need to talk about cases, and about problems in their work settings, such as disputes with colleagues or interdisciplinary conflicts. Often, they have little or no opportunity to talk either about any of these things except when they attend courses such as ours. We have come to realise that there is a conspicuous gap within primary care in this area and that we need to fill this gap by giving it a high profile on our courses. We have therefore come to think and talk of a style of clinical supervision that may accurately be described as 'narrative-based clinical supervision'.

We have also discovered that only a small minority of GPs (and an even smaller proportion of other professions such as primary care nurses, health visitors, pharmacists and optometrists) can commit themselves to a half-day course every week. We have therefore started to explore ways of offering a basic introduction to narrative-based clinical supervision in a variety of ways in other settings, including single study days around the UK and abroad, two- or three-day courses, or short seminars for GP registrars, new principals and trainers.

Narrative and primary care: the key ideas

Many psychologists nowadays argue that story-making is a fundamental part of being human. They claim that we all have a basic need to seek meaning and to give others an account of that meaning – in the form of stories or narratives. In the last few years, ideas about narratives have also become influential within the world of medicine. Whereas the idea that people need to 'construct' their stories, or their versions of reality, seemed a fairly abstruse idea to most doctors and health professionals a decade ago, it is now fairly commonplace. It is even possible to talk of a contemporary movement towards 'narrative-based medicine'. From a narrative-based perspective, every medical encounter may be seen as a collaborative attempt by a patient and a practitioner to construct an agreed story about what is going on (Launer 2002).

One way of looking at primary care is as a place where patients bring stories that contain puzzles, questions or things that do not yet make sense. They want professionals to try and help them to pull together a new and more coherent story. There may be a need for some practical and technical solutions, such as a prescription, injection or hospital referral. However, patients are unlikely to accept any advice or treatment unless it also makes sense as part of a new narrative.

If patients have a basic need to construct new stories, health professionals have the same need too. Telling anecdotes about cases is one crucial way that doctors create meaning out of what they do. Just as patients need to go away from consultations with stories that they feel they can recount to themselves and their families with new certainty and hope, professionals too need continual opportunities to reconstruct their own stories about what they do and what they achieve.

Patients' stories can get into a muddle, or hopelessly stuck. So can professional narratives. The practitioner who comes away from an encounter with a story of confusion, guilt or fear may be just as distressed as a patient with a similar predicament. Similarly, most tales of 'heartsink patients' are in reality tales of 'heartsink interactions' or of 'two heartsink story-tellers'. If patients come to professionals because they need to transform their stories into better ones, professionals also need such help. One definition of clinical supervision might be that it is an opportunity for a professional to change a story about a working encounter, by holding a conversation with another professional.

Conversations between professionals often serve to reinforce 'stuckness'. Professionals tend to use narratives to place themselves in a particular light, perhaps as heroes or victims, and to cast the other players in a more negative light, for example as adversaries. Such narratives often have a stereotypical quality about them. The characters are portrayed as unchangeable and the outcomes seem to be the only possible ones. Yet unless the professional can imagine alternative stories about the patient, the next encounter is unlikely to produce anything new. The task of a clinical supervisor might therefore be seen as challenging the supervisee to change stories that seem to be superficial, judgemental or unhelpful.

Not all the stories that professionals tell are about their patients. Many concern colleagues. Often, problematical stories about patients are linked to problematical stories about teams and professional networks. Helping professionals to explore better stories about their work with patients also involves helping them to think about their interactions with other professionals. It may be impossible for practitioners to change their narratives about cases until they can tell stories about their team-mates that are also less fixed and stereotypical.

One concept encapsulates the narrative approach: we all live and work within a web of interconnecting stories (Bruner 1990). Some of these stories are internal ones that we recite silently to ourselves in order to make sense of what we are doing. Others are stories that we hear or tell in conversations with patients and colleagues, relatives and friends. The stories constantly influence each other. They may reinforce elements of plot and character that are already established, or they may challenge these – so that next time the story is told in a different way. The stories that go on in our heads when we see patients are inseparably related to the stories that we tell colleagues about them afterwards – and to the stories we then tell to others concerning the colleagues themselves.

As an act of story-making, clinical supervision is inseparably linked both with reflective clinical practice and with effective teamwork. It suggests ways of generating more imaginative stories in consultations. It can propose more flexible and self-critical stories about working relationships. Clinical supervision can therefore be seen as a way of providing professionals with a chance to reflect on the story-making process itself, in all its different stages.

How we teach clinical supervision

In our teaching, we address supervision in a number of different ways.

- We demonstrate it in one-to-one interviews by the tutor, with the rest of the group observing.
- We ask group members to take turns at supervising each other on cases, by working in pairs, usually with one or more people observing them. We invite interviewers to take occasional breaks in order to hold a discussion with the observers: in effect to receive their own supervision.
- We encourage practitioners to create or explore opportunities for supervision of this kind in their workplace.

In order to get away from any idea of hierarchy or rank, we generally refer to 'interviewer' and 'interviewee' rather than supervisor and supervisee.

We teach a particular technique for clinical supervision, based on family therapy practice and supervision. This technique is sometimes known as 'interventive interviewing' but we prefer to use the description 'conversations inviting change'. The main idea is that properly structured conversations can lead to the production of a useful new story.

In contrast with the Balint approach, we promote an interviewing style based mainly on questioning. We believe that this helps interviewers to avoid becoming overinvolved or directive, and allows interviewees to have enough mental and emotional space to generate new ideas and solutions.

We also train interviewers to follow feedback constantly, by tracking the exact words and phrases used by practitioners, and making enquiries into these, for example: '*When you say you're confused about why he came, what are the different possibilities that go through your mind . . . ?*'

We particularly encourage interviewers to ask questions about the contexts surrounding the story. This usually involves seeking some understanding of who else is involved in the case apart from the practitioner being interviewed. It also involves a curiosity into the contexts surrounding the index patient: family, work colleagues, ethnic or cultural identity and so on, for example: '*Are there any areas of the patient's life that you might want to ask about, to shed light on what she's describing?*' The reason for this is that such questions often help practitioners to identify the gaps in their knowledge of the patient.

Interviewers can help by holding on to a view of the world as constituted from circular processes rather than linear ones. This means, for example, an ability to notice and draw attention to the effect the practitioner may be having on the patient and vice versa. It also means being alert to the iterative ways in which family members can intensify or modulate each other's stories.

Interviewers need to be neutral in relation to the story being presented. This means showing a non-judgemental attitude towards the practitioner and also to the patient being described. It also helps if the interviewer can stay neutral in relation to the 'facts' of the case, including the diagnosis, causes and so on, without showing a clear preference either for or against any of the particular descriptions or solutions being proposed.

One additional aspect of neutrality is in relation to theoretical beliefs: this means avoiding any fixed way of looking at the world (such as a psychoanalytic or psychiatric one) if this does not appear to be helping the practitioner. It means avoiding over-certain formulations, such as: '*Your patient sounds depressed*', and instead asking questions, such as: '*Did the patient use the word "depression"? Did you use it? What effect would it have if you suggested the word to your patient?*' and so on.

When people first practise this style of interviewing, they often say how they find it hard to maintain a neutral and questioning stance, particularly if the case is similar to one of their own. Learners also describe how they can feel stuck and uncertain in the early part of the interview – almost as if they have been infected by the interviewee's distress and inertia. However, with practice there is generally a big change in the interviewer's ability to ask imaginative questions. Most people also say that skills acquired through learning to conduct supervision in this way are useful as consulting skills in the everyday work of primary care. Indeed, many say that they find it easier to learn a narrative-based consulting style through supervising colleagues than they do by other means such as role play or analysis of videotaped consultations.

As for interviewees, they nearly always report how useful it is to have an independent person question them in a way that invites them so they can think new thoughts about cases that may have been upsetting, confusing or angering them.

Four frequently asked questions

Does this method work only in one-to-one interviews or can it be used in group discussions?

We have always found that the most effective way to teach narrative-based supervision is by using one-to-one interviews. So we generally break up any large group into groups of three or four people for intensive practice. One or more tutors then moves between the small groups, intervening as necessary to teach or reinforce the 'micro-skills' needed. Our overall objective is to help interviewees to 'change their story' and also to think of a repertoire of possible questions to ask their patients at the next consultation so the patients' story can also change. Our experience is that, when we work with the whole group, the discussion usually becomes too wide-ranging for this to happen. People too readily offer advice, or bring up different cases for comparison, instead of remaining neutral and questioning in their stance.

Another way we overcome this when teaching large groups is by putting the interviewer and practitioner in a 'fishbowl', with the rest of the group functioning as a 'reflecting team', invited to offer comments at intervals in the conversation, but in a structured way. On longer courses, a group working in this way can acquire sufficient skill and discipline to follow the ideas of interviewer and interviewee closely, and to ask appropriate questions rather than try and 'solve the problem'.

Is this kind of supervision only useful for psychosocial cases or can it be used for more medical ones?

There are no exclusions. In reality, GPs and primary care workers generally see few people who do not bring a mixture of physical and personal concerns. It can be artificial to try and set up distinctions or say what supervision can and cannot cover. If a supervisor or observer thinks it would be helpful to point out, for example, that a patient's cough might be caused by antihypertensive medication, it would be pointless to feel it was 'out or order' to mention it. The only proviso we suggest is that such information should always be offered in the form of a hypothesis (*'Do you think it's worth considering . . . ?'*) and not as a statement (*'Well it's probably because he's on enalapril'*).

What opportunities are there in everyday primary care to practise this kind of supervision?

This approach can be used in all kinds of ways and at all levels of skill. People who have attended a single afternoon's workshop have reported that it changed the way they subsequently offered help to their colleagues. Others have said that they are much readier to initiate conversations about their own cases with anyone who is available in their work setting. This might be a colleague from their own or another discipline, or with a medical student or registrar in the room ('*Can I tell you what's going on in this case and ask you to question me about it?*'). Practitioners who have studied the approach for a year or more will obviously be much more proficient in offering and receiving this kind of supervision, and they may also go out of their way to seek formal arrangements with a colleague for 'co-supervision'. However, there is no intrinsic reason why the method cannot be used, or adapted, for just about any case discussion between colleagues.

What do you do if case presenters indicate that they have underlying personal or professional problems?

Supervision is not the same as counselling or therapy, but clinical cases can have profound effects on practitioners – all the more so if they are themselves in a vulnerable state for any reason. Supervisors often have to tread a fine line between being too innocuous in their enquiries, and breaking down their colleagues' defences quite inappropriately. This is not an area where simple guidelines or recipe-book formulas can be offered, but some ideas seem to be helpful.

- There is nothing wrong with practitioners crying or sharing difficult memories if they wish to, and if they feel safe enough in the particular supervision setting.
- Supervisors should satisfy themselves – by constantly asking for feedback – that this really is what the interviewee wants and finds helpful at that moment.
- If the supervisor has any concern about the risk of unwanted overexposure, the case discussion should probably pause for some kind of 'discussion-about-the-discussion'. (For example: '*Is this conversation taking you into areas you'd rather not continue with for the moment?*' or '*If you felt this wasn't the ideal setting for looking into these issues, where else might you turn?*')

In a group teaching context, it may be entirely appropriate to approach interviewees privately at the end of the session to ask if they feel all right about what has taken place, and to offer the opportunity for a further confidential discussion – either with the interviewer or someone else.

An example

This 'case' illustrates a teaching session that took the form of a supervision interview. It has been drawn together from a number of different examples, in order to illustrate key points. All identifying details have been changed.

> Some time ago, a group of about 12 experienced GP trainers asked me to hold an all-day training session. They wanted to learn how to supervise their registrars on difficult cases more systematically. We spent the morning looking at the basic concepts and skills of narrative-based supervision. At the beginning of the afternoon, I asked if anyone had a clinical case from their own practice that was causing them concern and might benefit from supervision. Dr M said he had a case. I asked for another volunteer to carry out the supervision. Dr K came forward.

> With their agreement, I asked the two doctors to take their chairs into the centre of the room, with the rest of the group acting as observers. I said I would sit by Dr K, and might prompt her from time to time with some possible questions. I also explained that I might interrupt the interview to invite comments, hypotheses or questions from the rest of the group.

> Taking up some ideas from the morning's teaching, Dr K began not by asking Dr M to talk about the case, but by posing a few questions to help him to set the context: *'Is there anything we need to know about your practice or the way you work, to help us understand what is happening in this case . . . ?'*; *'Are you the only person currently involved in this case or do we need to know about any others . . . ?'*; *'Is this a case where we need to know about previous contacts with family members . . . ?'*; *'What was it about this case that made it spring to mind when the tutor asked for a volunteer just now?'*

> (**Commentary**: 'Contextualising' questions like this serve a number of purposes. They 'bond' the interviewer and interviewee in a non-threatening way. They establish important information that helps to make sense of the case – especially the kind of information that may get lost later on in a welter of factual content or strong emotion. They also invite the interviewee to start thinking about the case in a more reflective way and from an interactional perspective.)

> Dr M's case concerned someone that he had only seen for the first time the previous afternoon: a 15-year-old girl, Sandy, who was pregnant and unsure whether she wanted an abortion. From Dr M's answers to Dr K's opening questions, we learned a great deal that was relevant: for example, that Dr M worked in an inner city practice of four partners who were

willing to see 15-year-old girls in confidence and willing to refer patients for abortions. We also learned that the girl's mother, Karen, was single and was currently seeing one of Dr M's partners for a drug problem and depression. Apparently, what had brought the case to mind, and led Dr M to feel that supervision might be useful, was that the girl had seemed so casual. In spite of being nearly 12 weeks pregnant, she had seemed more concerned in the consultation to ask him to look at a clicky jaw that was bothering her. This put him, in his own words, 'off balance' in the consultation, and he felt he had not really conveyed the urgency he felt about her need to make a decision.

Once the interview had established these basics, I intervened to suggest to Dr K that she should ask Dr M to think of some hypotheses about Sandy's casualness, and about being caught 'off balance' by this. Talking about Sandy, Dr M said he thought she might be very scared but was 'testing him out'. Alternatively, it was possible that she was genuinely ignorant about pregnancy and abortions, and thought that there was lots of time to make a decision. Also, it could be that she was simply 'in denial'. He thought his own difficulties in the consultation were because he did not want to alienate her by pressure, or by second-guessing her decision. As a result, he felt he had had ended up too 'laid back' in his approach, and now felt cross both with himself and with Sandy.

(**Commentary**: Inviting hypotheses like this is generally a good way of inviting 'new stories' – not just single ones but multiple possible narratives. It invites interviewees to think of new perspectives and dimensions on the problems that are bothering them.)

After further questioning, Dr M said he felt that the likeliest explanation of Sandy's manner was that she was 'all over the place', unable to focus on anything except the relatively trivial or superficial, like the clicky jaw. He said she was due to see him again in three days, but he was now unsure how to help her take on board the seriousness of her predicament, or to help her to decide what to do.

I intervened to invite the other ten doctors present to offer ideas about further questions that Dr K could ask Dr M (or indeed that he could ask Sandy). Going round the circle, there was a richness of suggestions. People were interested in whether Sandy had disclosed the pregnancy to her mother, her boyfriend or anyone else. A lot of the doctors present wanted to know more about Sandy's current relationship with her mother, how Karen's drug habit and depression affected her, whether Sandy too might have the same problems, and whether she had any contact with her father. One person wondered if there was a teacher at school, or another trusted adult, that she could talk to. Was there anyone she might like to bring along to help her think about her pregnancy? A couple of people in the group were more curious about Dr M's own reaction: what did he fear might happen if he did actually spell out how serious things were, or asked her to think about what it would be like to have a baby – or to abort one?

(**Commentary**: Team discussions like this can be enormously productive of new ideas, but they can also overwhelm the person with the problem. For that reason, it is usually helpful for comments to be directed at the interviewer alone. The interviewee can sit back and listen – or tune out – as the various suggestions come up, selecting the ones that seem most helpful.)

Following the discussion, I helped Dr K to frame a series of questions to put to Dr M in order to round up the interview. These are the ones she decided to ask: '*What ideas have struck you most from this interview or the team discussion?*'; '*Are there any particular questions you now want to ask Sandy when you next see her?*'; '*How do you think you might deal with Sandy if she seems casual again, or if you feel you're getting too laid back, or cross?*'

Dr M reported that the interview had make him think a great deal. In particular, he felt he had a whole repertoire of questions to help Sandy take on board what was happening to her and think about how to deal with it. He also felt he was now equipped emotionally to steer a course between being avoiding the issue or being too harsh.

Conclusion

What we know from teaching narrative-based supervision, and evaluations of our teaching, is that it can help practitioners from many different disciplines to learn a new way of looking at cases. It can give them a new view of their own needs for supervision and support, and it offers an approach they can employ for themselves and their colleagues. For some, it can revolutionise their way of working and their understanding of primary care. However, one drawback of the method is that, while people readily appreciate the underlying concepts such as interventive interviewing and neutrality, they discover how difficult it can be to apply these in their everyday work without further skills, practice and training. There is a risk that, for some, a brief exposure to this method will lead them to feel relatively deskilled. Our task as tutors is therefore often to help people to integrate this approach into their existing ways of working, rather than to leave them feeling we have offered a 'gold standard' from which they will fall short. We also recognise that we have a wider task that is in some sense a cultural one: namely, to disseminate this kind of approach so that disciplined forms of peer and educational supervision become much more the norm in primary care.

Although we have good information regarding the effects on the practitioners we teach – in the form of their formal and informal feedback – we have no measures of any change that might be effected on their clinical performance. We do not know if their patients notice anything different or whether they like what they notice. We certainly do not know whether, at the end of the line, patient outcome improves as a result of practitioner training or practitioner supervision. We share these limitations with practically every other form of supervision and support currently on offer, but we also acknowledge that these are important issues that need to be addressed in the future.

References

Balint M (1957) *The Doctor, his Patient and the Illness.* Pitman, London.

Bruner J (1990) *Acts of Meaning.* Harvard University Press, Cambridge, MA.

Gosling R and Turquet P (1964) The training of general practitioners. In: R Gosling, D Miller, D Woodhouse and P Turquet (eds) *The Use of Small Groups in Training.* Codicote, London.

Launer J (2002) *Narrative-based Primary Care: a practical guide.* Radcliffe Medical Press, Oxford.

Launer J and Lindsey C (1997) Training for systemic general practice: a new approach from the Tavistock Clinic. *Br J Gen Prac.* 47: 453–6.

CHAPTER 9

Mentoring and co-tutoring

Paul Paxton and Paul Sackin

Introduction

In this chapter we propose to discuss a method of peer support for GPs that has been developed in East Anglia since 1994 and is known as 'co-tutoring'. We will explain what co-tutoring is, describe how it works using some examples, deal with some frequently asked questions about it and discuss its value. In the final part of the chapter we will compare and contrast our approach with mentoring, a method that may be more familiar to readers and which has a lot in common with co-tutoring.

How did co-tutoring start?

In 1994 Andrew Eastaugh, a GP in Suffolk, suggested co-tutoring as a process of mutual support and education. He saw it as a way of GPs becoming more 'collegiate'. The process could help with the isolation that many GPs were feeling at the time and could be a useful focus for the local Faculty of the Royal College of General Practitioners.

At the same time, and completely independently, Paul Paxton, a GP in Cambridge, also came up with an idea he called co-tutoring, intended as a means of enabling GPs to become more effective in their practice. He had noted how on many occasions participants on educational courses became enthusiastic about implementing new ideas in their practice, but on return to work lost this enthusiasm, and the impetus to make change happen. His belief was that with support and time for reflection GPs could deal with any blocks to making change happen.

Andrew Eastaugh set up the first course to introduce GPs to co-tutoring, and did so with the help of a colleague, Paul Sackin, an experienced medical educator and GP. At about the same time Paul Paxton assembled a group of people, including Paul Sackin, to plan a programme to introduce co-tutoring. From this planning the second course was developed and run by Paul Paxton and Marion

Barnett. A key factor in the success of the course was having a non-medical person as a facilitator (Marion Barnett) working alongside a GP facilitator. Following this course, which has become the basis for all future courses, it was decided to join the two separate efforts and work as a single team. Marion continued to facilitate subsequent courses along with Andrew Eastaugh, Paul Paxton or Paul Sackin. Sue Parlby took on the role of non-GP facilitator, also very successfully, after Marion became ill and sadly died.

The group of us discussed the underlying principles of co-tutoring in an editorial in the *British Journal of General Practice* (Sackin *et al.* 1997).

What is co-tutoring?

The main features of co-tutoring are as follows.

- It is a relationship between two or three people.
- The aim is to enable each other to become more effective in our professional lives, to identify where we want to get to, how that might be achieved and what blocks need to be overcome.
- It is based on the belief that we have the ability to solve our own problems given the right amount of support. In co-tutoring this support comes from aware, active listening with the listener giving complete respect for the speaker.
- It is mutual and non-hierarchical.
- It is a form of co-mentoring.
- The relationship is totally confidential (see 'Frequently asked questions' below).
- Co-tutoring can work in the short term but for full value it is best to work in a longer-term relationship with regular meetings.

The process of co-tutoring

- In a co-tutoring session the time is divided equally into half, or into thirds in the case of a trio. In a pair one person starts as speaker and the other listens, and at half-time the pair switch roles. In a trio each person will take a turn as speaker, listener and observer.
- Pairs or trios are encouraged to meet up at least once per month.
- The place of the meeting needs to be private and comfortable and there needs to be protected time.
- The listener is there to facilitate the speaker. Discussion or advice does not normally form part of the process. In a trio the third person acts as observer of the process and can give useful feedback.

- The process is one of active listening with skilled interventions. The interventions are to help the speaker towards a fuller understanding of a situation. Speakers identify their own agenda and are enabled to identify any blocks to change that are required.
- Being listened to with good attention can lead to the release of emotions. This can be helpful for overcoming blocks to thinking clearly, making decisions and acting on them. An example of this could be a situation whereby a person feels so angry about a situation he or she is unable to think past the anger. Once the anger has been expressed in a co-tutoring situation solutions are more likely to be found. This process will only happen if the speaker feels 'safe' enough for it to happen.
- To co-tutor successfully requires training in active listening with the use of skilled interventions, feedback and emotional awareness. Many doctors find that their wish to identify a 'diagnosis and management plan' can interfere with the listening required to co-tutor. This skill used every day in the consultation needs to be put aside in the co-tutoring context as the solutions are to come from the speaker. Interestingly, despite this different way of listening, one of the reported benefits of those doing co-tutoring is the improved listening happening in the consultation. Another block to listening is when listeners can identify with the content of the speaker's story and stop noticing where the speaker is getting stuck. Listeners need to have developed some emotional self-awareness and ability to handle their own emotions in order to enable the speaker to identify and deal with emotions arising in the co-tutoring session. If a listener had a difficulty in dealing with their own or someone else's anger it is likely that the speaker would be aware of this and avoid dealing with their own anger in a co-tutoring session.

Active listening with skilled interventions, feedback skills and emotional awareness are all addressed in the introductory co-tutoring course which is a two-day residential one followed up by two one-day workshops three and nine months later.

Frequently asked questions

How are the pairs chosen?

This frequent question probably reflects a commonly shared fear of not being chosen, for example for team sports at school or at the disco. The system now evolved in the introductory course is to engage the participants in an exercise to work out what the advantages and disadvantages might be of working with someone that they are not immediately attracted to as well those that they are.

Working with someone one is not initially attracted to can overcome the development of a collusive relationship. This exercise comes towards the end of the course by which time everyone will have had opportunities to work in pairs with each other. The participants are then asked to write down the names of those they could work with in order of preference. They are encouraged to write down as many names as possible. These lists are kept confidential to the group and handed in to the facilitators who will then choose the pairs or trios.

What about confidentiality?

The relationship is a confidential one. If the pair meet outside their co-tutoring session it would not be appropriate for the listener to ask about an issue arising from the speaker's agenda unless the speaker chose to raise it.

What happens if one co-tutor becomes depressed or has an addiction?

Some concern has been expressed about the duty of a doctor if, as the listener, it becomes apparent that a speaker is at significant risk to himself or to patients. Although this is a highly unlikely scenario, what then should the listener do? Clearly, the best outcome would be for the listener to encourage the speaker to take appropriate action and preserve the relationship. If the speaker were not willing to seek help then the listener would be forced to break confidence and alert the appropriate bodies.

Can it be used for revalidation?

Not directly, although it can be used to support the process. The strength of the relationship is that it is non-judgemental and not an assessment of each other's abilities. This allows for greater honesty in disclosing difficulties and mistakes.

Is it co-counselling?

No. There are significant differences but some similarities. 'Co-counselling' as defined in Re-evaluation Counselling™ (Jackins 1965, 1982) has a different purpose and method. The purpose of Re-evaluation Counselling is to free each other of the distresses and hurts of the past, many of which are of societal origin, for example dependent on race, class, sexuality, gender, etc. The method used is that of emotional discharge (release), such as crying, laughing, shaking, etc. Although emotions may be expressed in a co-tutoring session, and when this happens it is encouraged, it is not the main purpose of the interaction. Similarities between co-tutoring and co-counselling include the paired structure, the equal sharing of time and some of the beliefs, for example the fact that individuals can sort out their own difficulties with good support. Both share a humanistic viewpoint. Some of the co-tutoring facilitators are also co-counsellors. This has provided some extra safety for the group when emotions have been expressed.

Can it work between doctor and non-doctor?

Yes. However, many doctors prefer to work with other doctors. This is partly due to feeling safe enough to talk about some medical stories, perhaps with unpleasant details, without fear of upsetting the listener. There is also the belief expressed by some participants that the listener needs to understand the medical details in order to be a co-tutor. This is not so. Sometimes being too involved with the content can actually hinder effective listening. Many doctors find it very difficult to notice the process involved in an interaction and focus instead on the content.

How do you deal with problems of avoidance or collusion and how do you get help if it goes wrong?

The main way of dealing with this is attendance at follow-up workshops. At the workshops participants identify areas of co-tutoring that are going well, in addition to those areas that they are finding hard. The day is spent working on participants' agendas and identifying ways of dealing with the problems encountered in the co-tutoring process. One of the methods used on the day is 'coached co-tutoring'. A co-tutoring pair works in front of the group with the support of the facilitators, one facilitator supporting the speaker and the other the listener. Any of the four can stop the proceedings at any time to look at how the process is going.

All co-tutors can ask for supervision from one or more of the facilitators. This option has only occasionally been taken up, although it has always proved very helpful.

What are the main problems people have experienced in co-tutoring?

The most common difficulty has been that of finding enough time to meet regularly. Some have tried to meet more informally, for example in a pub, and this has not proved helpful. Some have found it difficult to stick to sharing the time equitably between each other.

A co-tutoring vignette

This is a co-tutoring session between Drs B and J. We think it is reasonably typical but for obvious reasons it is fictitious. Dr B is the listener and the session started about five minutes earlier. Dr B summarises Dr J's agenda.

B: *'You've mentioned some difficulties that you have with your practice manager, and some problems you have with overrunning in your surgeries. Which one would you like to look at first?'*

J: *'I think I want to look at the second as it causes me most pressure . . .'*

B: *'Do you want to tell me what that the pressure is like?'*

J: *'Well I feel tense. In fact I already feel tense even before I get to the surgery. I am already thinking about being behind even before I start! Sometimes I know that because I'm tense I actually arrive late because I faff around at home trying to find things and make sure the kids are ready for school. I even feel tense talking about this now!'* [laughs]

B: *'OK, so what happens when you do get started seeing patients?'*

J: *'I listen well and patients seem to like coming to see me, they certainly talk! I get a lot of tears and as you know that takes time . . . and tissues. Then I think two things happen. I suddenly realise that the consultation has already gone on longer than it should and I interrupt to try and finish it. This causes a further lengthening as the patient eventually comes back to what they were saying before my interruption. The effect of my interruption is just to add more time on. The second thing that happens is when I think the consultation is at an end the patient brings up another problem they want dealing with. A good example was yesterday when I saw X. She came in and started talking about her bereavement. She became quite tearful. I gave her plenty of time and after about 20 minutes, when I was just finishing the consultation, or so I thought, she mentioned a change in her bowel habit. I suddenly felt really anxious but knew I had to deal with this as well. By the time I finished the whole thing had taken 40 minutes! I had three more patients to see afterwards and I know that because I felt pressured I tried to rush them and cut corners and became even more inefficient.'*

B: *'You sound very clear about the problem . . .'*

J: *'Well, yes and as I've talked it's become a lot clearer to me. It's quite a relief talking about it. [a sigh followed by laughter] I also recognise that part of my tension is because of Dr S in the practice who is really quite critical about me over-running. In fact I feel quite angry with him, as it is often his patients who come to see me saying that they find me easier to talk to!' [more laughter]*

B: *'Well recognised. So, what are your next steps in dealing with all of this?'*

J: *'I think that firstly I need to get myself sorted out at home. In fact I need to discuss this with my partner so that we can be more organised with the children. It would make such a difference just starting my surgery on time. I also think I could go on a consultation skills course but . . . that would be harder . . .'*

B: *'So, what would be hard about that?'*

The session continues with J exploring her fears about attending a consultation skills course.

Does co-tutoring work?

The basis of co-tutoring is the empowerment given to participants by skilled and supportive listening. This empowerment is a subjective process so that anecdotal accounts of the effectiveness of co-tutoring are important evidence for its success. Many participants attest to the help they have had from co-tutoring. Some would regard it as having helped them to change their lives, perhaps to give them the courage (for example) to move to a more congenial general practice partnership. Many others report less dramatic but very useful outcomes. The common theme is one of support and empowerment, enabling them to move forward in their professional and personal lives in ways that they feel would not have been possible without the help of their co-tutor(s).

Hibble and Berrington (1998) provide some objective evidence for the effectiveness of co-tutoring. These authors sent a questionnaire to East Anglian GPs who were involved in mentoring or co-tutoring, as well as a control group involved in neither. Fifty-two per cent of the co-tutoring group had defined and recorded personal development plans compared to 26% of the mentoring group and 13% of the control group. The co-tutoring group also reported a greater reduction in stress than either of the other groups.

A more detailed, qualitative evaluation of co-tutoring has been carried out by McKee and Norris (1999a, b). These authors looked in detail at one of the London groups of co-tutors and also a few of the more experienced East Anglian co-tutors. As well as reviewing relevant literature, these researchers' methods included semi-structured interviews of participants and facilitators and direct observation of co-tutoring pairs and trios and of training days. Some key observations of the researchers were that:

- co-tutoring incorporates both therapeutic and educational type responses to experience, offering the possibility of recovering and learning from experience
- despite, perhaps because of, a wide-angled lens approach to content, some of the outcomes from co-tutoring are focused on clinical skills and healthcare management
- the most frequently cited outcome was an improvement in consulting skills
- co-tutoring was identified as having provided motivation and support to sustain GPs in their (wider) professional role (most London co-tutors were active in setting up their PCGs)
- the willingness to look after their co-tutoring partners, should they become depressed or 'ill', suggests that co-tutoring might provide an alternative or supplementary service to the sick doctor scheme.

(The co-tutoring facilitators would not see this last point as appropriate in co-tutoring. This raises important boundary issues. A co-tutor is not a doctor or therapist for their co-tutoring partner. Should someone become too depressed to give as well as receive in the relationship, that is, 'two-way', the role of the other would be to be supportive and encourage appropriate help from elsewhere rather than slip into a therapeutic 'one-way' relationship.)

How has co-tutoring evolved and what are the challenges?

Since 1994 there have been 12 introductory co-tutoring courses, mainly in East Anglia, but also in London and in Newcastle upon Tyne. Thus, approximately 150 people have taken up co-tutoring and many are still engaged in it. In addition, we have run many workshops throughout the country that have given people a taste of co-tutoring. As a result the ideas have received considerable publicity and no doubt have been taken up by some people even if they are not fully engaged in the process.

One of the challenges we face is making co-tutoring appear more relevant to a wider group. Co-tutoring could be invaluable, for example, in helping GPs to prepare for appraisal and revalidation, as well as for developing their personal learning plans. Yet we feel that attendance at an introductory course is essential for obtaining the necessary skills. This may be seen as too great an investment in time (and sometimes money) for many GPs.

We have found that some of the more recent co-tutoring groups have had a relatively high drop-out rate. This has been partly due to unavoidable difficulties, such as one co-tutor moving away or the co-tutoring pair living a long way away from each other. But perhaps there is a more fundamental difficulty. There is no doubt that, at least in the early stages, co-tutoring pairs or trios find it hard to recapture the depth of work achieved in the introductory course. They seem to need much more time and opportunity to practise the skills that they have started to learn. We are looking at ways to address this problem. One solution might be to offer an alternative version of co-tutoring that consists relatively more of group meetings with facilitators than of meetings of the individual pairs and trios.

Mentoring

The concept of mentoring derives from Mentor in Homer's *Odyssey*. Mentor was charged with supporting and guiding Telemachus, the son of Odysseus, while his father was away fighting the Trojan wars. From these early beginnings mentoring has come to mean different things in different contexts and professions (Freeman 1998) but the concept of support being offered by somebody older and wiser usually holds.

A number of different mentoring schemes have developed in general practice in recent years (Alliott 1996; Freeman 1998). These have differed in detail but most have had in common support given by a mentor to a doctor's learning. Mentoring is seen as an integral element of portfolio-based learning (RCGP 1993). This method, derived from the graphic arts, is a form of self-directed learning involving the collection of evidence (the portfolio) that learning has taken place. The Royal College of General Practitioners (RCGP) took up portfolio-based learning enthusiastically in the 1990s and it has been an important stage in the evolution of current ideas for personal learning plans and revalidation folders. 'The process of building the portfolio benefits from the assistance of a "mentor" who enables and facilitates it' (learning) (RCGP 1993). The RCGP occasional paper goes on to describe several stages of portfolio-based learning in which the mentor is involved. These stages include identifying the learning experience, reflecting on it, identifying new learning needs and devising a plan to meet them.

Some mentoring schemes are more broadly based and offer 'pastoral' support as well as help with learning. Alliott (1996) describes schemes such as facilitatory mentoring. Arguably, the skills required by these 'generic' mentors are very similar to those used in the listening role of co-tutoring.

How, then, do mentoring and co-tutoring compare? Co-tutoring is a particular form of co-mentoring, a term used for those mentoring each other. Co-tutoring arguably has the advantage of being completely non-hierarchical. Participants of varying age and experience can learn equally from each other. Co-tutors are invariably both facilitators and learners, whereas mentors are only involved with facilitation.

Proctor (2000) has described three desirable functions of supervision. The 'formative' function, to do with personal development, is likely to be well served by both mentoring and co-tutoring. Arguably, the 'restorative' function, to do with support, is better served by the close and long-term relationship that obtains in co-tutoring. On the other hand the 'normative' function, to do with quality, will be an integral part of the mentoring that accompanies portfolio-based learning but may not always feature so much in co-tutoring or in more pastoral forms of mentoring.

Mentoring and co-tutoring can exist happily together. Co-tutoring skills can be used by mentors and, indeed, mentors can receive support for themselves by using the co-tutoring process. Some co-tutors have used a mentor to help with a particular aspect of their learning while continuing to co-tutor. Some people may prefer not to engage in the skills of co-tutoring but would like to have the support of a mentor. Others may be more comfortable in a more hierarchical situation. There may be practical issues to consider in setting up mentoring or co-tutoring schemes that may make one a more viable arrangement in a particular area than another. There is no doubt that the training for both mentoring and co-tutoring have a great deal in common and we have contributed to the development of several mentoring schemes in England.

Conclusion

Co-tutoring formalises and extends supportive, mentoring relationships between peers. It has been shown that such relationships can enhance learning (Goodlad 1995). Co-tutoring has made a considerable impact on many of its participants. It is a powerful method of support and it can be used as a non-hierarchical form of supervision in primary care.

References

Alliott R (1996) Facilitatory mentoring in general practice. *BMJ (Career Focus)*. **28 September**: 2–3.

Freeman R (1998) *Mentoring in General Practice*. Butterworth–Heinemann, Oxford.

Goodlad S (ed.) 1995 *Students as Tutors and Mentors*. Kogan Page, London.

Hibble A and Berrington R (1998) Personal professional learning plans – an evaluation of mentoring and co-tutoring in general practice. *Educ Gen Pract.* **9**: 216–21.

Jackins H (1965) *The Human Side of Human Beings.* Rational Island Publishers, Seattle.

Jackins H (1982) The art of listening. In: H Jackins (ed.) *The Fundamentals of Co-counselling Manual.* Rational Island Publishers, Seattle.

McKee A and Norris N (1999a) *Making Experience Educational – co-tutoring, peer facilitated learning. Final Report.* Centre for Applied Research in Education, University of East Anglia, Norwich.

McKee A and Norris N (1999b) *Making Experience Educational – co-tutoring, peer facilitated learning. Executive Summary, Final Report.* Centre for Applied Research in Education, University of East Anglia, Norwich.

Proctor B (2000) Training for the supervision alliance attitude, skills and intention. In: J Cutcliffe, T Butterworth and B Proctor (eds) *Fundamental Themes in Clinical Supervision.* Blackwell, Oxford.

RCGP Working Group on Higher Professional Education (1993) *Portfolio-based Learning in General Practice.* Occasional paper 63. Royal College of General Practitioners, London.

Sackin P, Barnett M, Eastaugh A and Paxton P (1997) Peer-supported learning. *Br J Gen Prac.* **47**: 67–8.

Further details

Co-tutoring is administered by the East Anglia Faculty of the Royal College of General Practitioners. For further details and to contact us, please visit our website (www.co-tutoring.org).

CHAPTER 10

Peer supervision groups: a delicate but powerful process

*Steve Hiew, Nalliah Sivananthan and
Jonathan Burton*

Background

The north London boroughs of Enfield and Haringey extend radially from a socially deprived, multi-ethnic inner city to the affluent, leafy suburbs bordered by the M25. Since the early 1990s there has been a culture of grassroots organisations in primary care in the district, including GP forums, community nurse forums and practice manager forums. These proliferated particularly between 1995 and 1998, when a regional initiative 'Development Through Education' (also known as the LIZEI programme) provided support for protected time for learning. One aspect of this grassroots movement was the development of self-directed learning groups across parts of Enfield and Haringey.

How these groups developed

The self-directed learning group movement was led by local health professionals. Originally, this movement was for GPs only but multiprofessional groups arose subsequently in some areas. For example, healthcare professionals working in one locality were invited to join a closed group. Members met monthly at a local community nurses' clinic or GP surgery (Hiew and Sivananthan 2001). Up to 14 groups have been documented (Burton 1998) in Enfield and Haringey (north central London). As groups do, some have dispersed while new ones have formed. The longest-established group has survived for nine years. Of the 14 groups noted in 1998, six were multiprofessional, each group having anything up to 20 members.

In Chapter 1 (page 4), supervision was defined as '*facilitated learning in relation to live practical issues*'. In fact, the origins of the self-directed learning groups lay in the concerns of various professional groups for action over exactly such problems. Historically, the groups arose out of local doctors' forums, the purpose of which was to discuss the real, live and practical issues of daily practice. The forums were action groups rather than learning groups. This history was a very important context for the self-directed learning groups, because members had already become accustomed to meeting to discuss their concerns. The self-directed learning groups therefore added structure, safety and a commitment to going beyond discussion to learning.

The leaders of self-directed learning groups were themselves very often untrained as educators. In some way this may have been an advantage as it enabled them to come together with a fresh view as to what might or might not work in the very environment that they understood and concerning the problems which they and their colleagues faced on a daily basis. The leaders were responsible for maintaining the shape and cohesion of the group, and for administering its activities, but the groups were set up so that the supported learning took place in a peer setting and through peer influence.

Tools

Together, the groups have developed and refined a number of tools, in order to create a safe environment for peer learning and to ensure that continuity and values are prime considerations for group members. The main tools for self-directed learning groups are as follows.

Ground rules

These lay out the behaviour to be followed by group members, to ensure they do not inhibit each other. Important points include confidentiality, mutual respect and commitment to learning rather than criticism. (*See* Box for a sample list.)

Sample list of ground rules from a typical self-directed learning group

- Safe environment paramount
- All are equal
- Everyone is a teacher as well as a learner
- Focus to improve quality, not to find faults
- Reflect on proceedings, document decisions
- Commit to self-evaluation
- Preserve materials in personal portfolio

S D L ENCOUNTER FORM

Name S. Omeone   Position Practice Nurse
Address 123 Palace Rd, London N22
Institution The Sandy Park Surgery

What was your encounter?
e.g.   Patient episode? Reading? Lecture? Video? Mass media? Hearsay?
A brief description of the encounter
A relative of mine asked me about screening for prostate cancer,
because a newspaper article advocated screening in younger men.

What was your concern?
e.g.   Diagnosis? Prognosis? Treatment? Effectiveness? Patient acceptance?
Is the test accurate? Are younger men at risk?

How did you try to find answers?
e.g.   Ask a colleague? Looked up library/internet? Attend a course?
Looked up publication (Effective Healthcare Bulletin).

Were the answers you found backed by sound evidence?
Article contained references to original research (screening is
not worthwhile).
Checked with local Public Health dept – confirmed news report
is controversial.

Has this encounter made any impact on your patient care?
e.g.   Improved knowledge? Changed attitude? Changed behaviour?
Improved knowledge.
Also became more aware of effect of mass media and their
limited accuracy.

How will you share your learning with your team members?
Discuss problem and finding during practice meeting.
Add copy of publication to practice library.

©1998 Dr Sivananthan & Hiew

Figure 10.1   The self-directed learning encounter form.

Encounter form

This is a data collection instrument (Figure 10.1) used by individual participants to record any significant events in their daily professional lives. An 'event' might be one that raised clinical doubts or caused much impact. The practitioner also records on the form how he/she dealt with it, and the sources of information used.

Acceptance of the 'three circle' concept

This is derived from the 80/20 principle (Koch 1999), which shows how in all human endeavours there will be consensus, controversy and dissent. On average, consensus will include 80% of individuals, whereas 20% of individuals will be doubters or dissenters (although obviously these proportions may vary greatly from occasion to occasion). Individuals in the consensus group can learn from the minority doubters or dissenters and vice versa, as long as all are listened to.

Reflective evaluation form

This is a set of prompts to be completed at the end of each session in order to record relevant ideas and action plans. The group reviews these at the beginning of the subsequent session and any deviations are recorded in individuals' portfolios.

Portfolio

This is made up of encounter forms, notes of discussions, copies of evidence (*see below*) and reflective evaluation forms. Physically, the portfolio was a green ring binder. All members have their own and most keep them for personal reference. They could, of course, form the basis of portfolios for appraisal and re-accreditation.

Agenda setting

At the start of each meeting, members reflect on the decisions from the previous meeting and whether they had followed them through, using their portfolios. The subsequent agenda for each meeting is set by the group; it is based on the encounter forms of one or two of them.

Further resources

Whenever an encounter has generated a clinical question that cannot be answered by other group members, the leader encourages participants to seek evidence in the scientific literature. Additional support is offered in the form of advice on appropriate sources. Sometimes the search is done on their behalf. This may be at libraries in local healthcare trusts, on the internet, or from collections of publications, such as *Effective Healthcare* and *Bandolier*.

Values

Groups thrive on shared values. They do not succeed if they feel they are assembled to carry through someone else's bidding. When trying to establish shared values, it helps to define the purer reasons for meeting as a group. In helping others set up similar groups, we often start by defining the importance of shared values: the duty to learn and the pleasure of learning together may be encapsulated in the following motto: 'Seek to understand, strive to be understood.'

Two encounters

Here are two examples of encounters and how they were dealt with in a self-directed learning group.

Encounter 1

S, a practice nurse, encountered her uncle in a supermarket. He asked her opinion about a screening test for prostate cancer, prostate specific antigen (PSA), which he had read in a magazine. S bluffed but felt uncomfortable, and realised that she could be asked the same again by patients attending her clinic. She consulted the GP she worked with, who was also embarrassed to have no answer. After open discussion in the group, they looked up the *Effective Healthcare* bulletin. They found the advice was provided in a professionals' version and a patients' version. The finding was taken back to the practice. At the long-term review (*see below*), S recalled that one year later an old man did come to ask about PSA. She gave him the patients' leaflet and the man decided for himself whether to have the test.

Encounter 2

In the 1990s, fresh doubts were cast over the MMR vaccine. Newspapers described the possibility of developing Crohn's disease in later life, and parents flooded GPs, practice nurses and health visitors with enquiries. Group members became concerned by the effect this had on immunisation uptake, and the lack of immediate clear guidance from the government, the scientists and drug companies. One GP decided to telephone the Royal Free Hospital for clarification of the evidence, and was met with silence. In the end the group members agreed to give out the same message to all patients. They realised that (i) patients tell each other what their doctors say; (ii) health visitors and community nurses were just as isolated as single-handed GPs, despite being in a big organisation; (iii) all practitioners in the area need to be aware of changing issues.

Two practitioners

Here are two accounts of the experiences of particular practitioners.

Dr Z: confidentiality and mutual respect

Dr Z attended meetings for five months without speaking up. In the sixth month, he asked if he could share an encounter from several months ago. This was about a child who developed a non-specific rash, fever and cervical lymph nodes. Unfortunately, the patient later died from Kawasaki disease and an inquiry was held against Dr Z. He had read about the condition and found little that could have helped earlier diagnosis. However, the data suggested that the disease was becoming more common in Western countries. Having gained confidence about the group, he was able to share his grief and educate everyone else. The experience was uplifting to everyone and a threat was turned into an opportunity. Dr Z remained an active member of the group afterwards.

Dr K: listening to and learning from the minority view

Dr K, who had extensive experience in psychiatry, suggested the use of small doses of diazepam (Valium) to treat anxiety. He explained that patients with anxiety suffer far more than those with depression or schizophrenia. Eight of the ten people present thought he was out of date and benzodiazepines should be avoided. However, they respected his experience and the meeting broke up with people agreeing to differ. Many months later, one of the ten GPs, Dr A, encountered a patient who was disabled by anxiety symptoms. Although Dr A had been in the anti-Valium camp, she recalled Dr K's experience and decided to try her patient on a small dose of diazepam. A few weeks later, the patient returned to tell Dr A that the tablets had helped her sort out the problems that caused her anxiety, and she had stopped taking them.

Discussion

Learning groups in primary care have been described for more than 20 years (Leeuwenhorst European Working Party 1980). It is recognised that groups provide individuals with support and motivation (Spurrell 1999). They serve to break down professional isolation. The building of trusting relationships is widely mentioned as an important outcome of the group experience. In areas like Enfield and Haringey, where many doctors practise single-handed with minimal ancillary staff, this was particularly pertinent. Unpublished evaluations of the Enfield and Haringey experiments of the 1990s have been undertaken, including the unpublished work of Stella Phillipps (*The Self Directed Learning Programme in Enfield and Haringey – an executive summary based on research evidence*). These have been based on interviews with participants. Practitioners have rated the comfortable environment and trusting relationships formed in the group as its most important aspect. Many commentaries on self-directed learning groups for health professionals in the literature (Dennick and Exley 1998; Peloso and Stakiw 2000) emphasise the power of the peer group to influence and mould the behaviour and attitudes of its members and to lead to episodes of significant learning (Eliasson and Mattson 1999). Members of the Enfield and Haringey groups have reported personal change in attitudes or behaviour. For example, they have reported an increased adoption of evidence-based clinical practice, an increased ability to handle uncertainty, to reduce management risk, and to find ways of dealing with patient demands and issues of public faith.

What other influences may be attributed to these groups? The format of the Enfield and Haringey learning groups was widely admired, as it was a unique grassroots movement which took place in an unfashionable area and among professionals who had never before been in the limelight. The success of this learning and support movement became known throughout the regional educational network. It gave heart to others to start similar movements which still survive (Herbert 2002). Some of the unique aspects of the groups also crossed into other settings. Nurses who had participated in the multiprofessional groups felt the encounter form (Figure 10.1) so useful that they had brought it into use with their own students.

A lot of emotional energy goes into sustaining a self-directed learning group and, not surprisingly, the groups in Enfield and Haringey had almost all ceased to exist by 2002. Difficulties in sustaining self-directed learning groups are common (Eliasson and Mattson 1999) unless there is a reason why members should go on attending. For example, attendance at the group may be the decreed method through which professional development takes place, as now happens with psychiatrists in the UK. The practical and emotional efforts of being a group leader also represent an area of vulnerability for such groups. Clearly, group leaders need support and supervision themselves.

Finding out what you did not know you did not know is one of the most important aspects of being supervised. The self-directed learning group provides a mechanism for this to happen. Sitting and talking about cases with people who do the same sort of job as you do, in a structured setting, provides ample opportunity for discovery and change. Previous descriptions of group learning have emphasised the peer group approach as empowerment for change (Dennick and Exley 1998; Hartmann 1995; Morris *et al.* 2001).

The model described here is different in that it allows dissent but this also leads to behaviour change. This delicate but powerful process is facilitated by customised tools. The importance of valuing the individual experience has been noted by Brookfield (1991). Individual contributions, especially if based on minority views, also serve to dispel a group's tendency to what is known as 'confirmation bias':

> groups often come to assume that all members think the same way ... an environment that does not encourage contributions also increases confirmation bias, where the majority seek information consistent with their beliefs and theories. (Sweet 1999)

We see the 80/20 rule (Koch 1999) as creating a safe 'demilitarised zone' that assists conflict resolution between individuals and maintains group integrity. However, it also permits sceptical individuals to remain open-minded, to think and make their own discoveries.

Many readers working in primary care will recognise from their own experience that learning groups have the potential for providing a peer supervision experience, by allowing peer-facilitated learning in relation to live practical issues. Clearly, how the group works, how group leaders are supported, how safe it feels for individuals, how much it offers opportunities for change – these are all key issues. Other self-directed groups work in different ways, so the tools which are described here are not the *sine qua non* of success, but they do illustrate an approach that ensured that significant learning did occur in respect of live practical issues and which offered support to group members.

References

Brookfield S (1991) *Understanding and Facilitating Adult Learning.* Open University Press, Milton Keynes.

Burton J (1998) Multipractice, selfdirected learning groups in North Thames East Region. *Educ Gen Pract.* **9**: 512–17 (Supplement).

Dennick R and Exley K (1998) Teaching and learning in groups and teams. *Biochem Ed.* **26**: 111–15.

Eliasson G and Mattson B (1999) From teaching to learning. Experiences of small CME group work in general practice in Sweden. *Scand J Prim Care.* **17**: 196–200.

Hartmann P (1995) Effects of peer-review groups on physicians' practice. *Eur J Gen Pract.* **1**: 107–12.

Herbert P (2002) The practice tutor scheme in Camden and Islington and South Barnet. *J Learn Work.* **4**: 7–9. (www.tlw.org.uk)

Hiew S and Sivananthan N (2001) The partnership in progress in practice project. *J Learn Work.* **3**: 6–10. (www.tlw.org.uk)

Koch R (1999) *The 80/20 Principle.* Doubleday, New York.

Leeuwenhorst European Working Party (1980) Continuing education and general practitioners. *Medical Education.* **14**: 227–8.

Morris P, Burton K, Reiss M and Burton J (2001) The difficult consultation. An action learning project about mental health issues in the consultation. *Educ Gen Pract.* **11**: 19–26.

Peloso P and Stakiw K (2000) Small group learning format for continuing medical education: a report from the field. *J Cont Ed Health Profess.* **20**: 27–32.

Spurrell M (1999) Consultant learning groups in psychiatry: report on a pilot study. *Psychiatric Bulletin.* **24**: 390–2.

Sweet T (1999) Special brew. *Health Service Journal.* **109**: 56–7.

PART IV

Supervision in GP training: fitting the realities

CHAPTER 11

Higher professional education for GPs: will this change the culture?

Tareq Abouharb and Neil Jackson

Glossary of terms

ADPGPE	Associate Dean of Postgraduate General Practice Education	Works under DsPGPE with specific brief for education and training
COGPED	Committee of General Practice Education Directors	National Committee
Deanery		Regional organisations to oversee GP education
DsPGPE	Director of Postgraduate General Practice Education	In charge of above
GP Registrar		Doctor during his or her apprentice year in general practice
HImP	Health Improvement Programme	Local health programme
HPE	Higher Professional Education	Post-vocational training for GPs
NSF	National Service Framework	Quality programme for management of diabetes, heart disease, cancer, etc.

New GP		During the first two years after completing vocational training
Non-principal		Independent GP, usually a locum
PCT	Primary Care Trust	NHS organisation for primary care services
Principal		Independent GP with list of patients and contractual responsibilities
PD	Programme Director	Educators for HPE scheme
SHA	Strategic Health Authority	New health authorities created in 2002
PDP	Personal Development Plan	Learning plan based on learning needs evaluation
VTS	Vocational Training Scheme	Training scheme for general practice. Three-year programme with one year in general practice, two years in hospital

Introduction

The concept of higher professional education (HPE) for newly qualified GPs has been established for a number of years. HPE may be considered as the provision of additional supervision and support to help newly qualified GPs in the transition from GP registrar to established independent practice as a GP principal or non-principal. It is now generally accepted that this provision should be given for at least a two-year period after completion of basic vocational training.

The background, development and facilitating of HPE will be discussed within this chapter in the setting of supervision and support, both on a one-to-one level and in the group situation. We hope to show that the structure offered by this method can prove helpful to delivering the educational needs of new GPs.

Background

The Royal College of General Practitioners (RCGP 1965) recommended that GP vocational training should take place over a four-year period, thus emphasising the need for an appropriate length of training period with adequate supervision and support to prepare young doctors for the realities of their future working lives in general practice.

Despite this, the NHS General Practice Vocational Training Regulations (which were established in 1979) specified that three years' full-time employment (or part-time equivalent) were required to satisfy the Regulations for prescribed experience. The three years would be made up of one year as a trainee general practitioner (GP registrar) and the remainder in hospital posts in fields which were considered appropriate for general practice training.

By the early 1990s it had become apparent that GPs were expected to fulfil an expanding role in the NHS. They needed to be adequately equipped for this new kind of job. It was realised that the basic three-year programme of GP vocational training could not be sufficient for the modern-day GP. If the three-year envelope for GP training was to remain intact, there was then a need to establish a system of post-vocational training support in the form of an agreed framework for higher professional education.

The evidence base for HPE

In 1998 the Committee of General Practice Education Directors (COGPED) published its report on HPE (Jackson and Reiss 1998). The prevailing view, expressed in this report, was that many recently vocationally trained GP registrars would benefit from an additional one or two years of supervision and support in a suitable learning environment. This would increase their preparedness and fitness for their role through a number of approaches, for example:

- enhancing the development of research and teaching skills
- undertaking a masters degree course or similar higher qualification
- developing additional clinical skills
- enhancing information technology and management skills
- generally heightening awareness of the role of GPs in the wider primary care context, including the complexities of the enhanced role of GPs in providing and commissioning care for patients.

The important issue identified in the report was the provision of ongoing educational support at the start of a new GP's career to enhance both competence and confidence. Also, the report noted that although progress was being made in the provision of HPE for new GPs, with a variety of educational initiatives in different parts of the UK, there was a lack of a proper financial framework for making educational support available. This lack was impeding progress and further development.

The report also highlighted various aspects of what was thought to be the appropriate educational context of HPE. These included:

- learner-centredness
- personal learning plans
- the provision of mentoring
- peer group support
- multiprofessional or multidisciplinary working.

The final report (NHS Executive 1998) of the London Initiative Zone Educational Incentive (LIZEI) scheme was also published in 1998. This three-year programme of educational initiatives for general practice from 1995 to 1998 was set within a framework of the four 'Rs', that is, Recruitment, Retention, Refreshment and Reflection. The scheme itself offered many varied training opportunities. One of these, the London Academic Training Scheme (LATS) (Freeman 1997), is an excellent example of an HPE initiative. It offers an additional period of 12 months' academic training with support through a facilitated group for GP registrars after completion of the basic GP vocational training programme.

Also in 1998 an influential report was published (Joint Centre for Education in Medicine 1998). This highlighted the problems with the transition from GP registrar to GP principal and an associated sudden reduction in educational supervision and support after completion of vocational training. The report illustrated the reluctance of newly qualified GPs to enter a principal post. It suggested that this cohort of doctors had further training needs. It recognised that there was a largely unstructured approach to facilitating their further training and development, without properly organised educational supervision and support.

Was this a problem primarily stemming from the length and educational content of the GP vocational training programme, which was not sufficient preparation for the new GP principal? If the vocational training programme was to be extended, what of the content and process of learning? Should it be more of the same or something entirely different? On the other hand, could it be that the basic vocational training programme was sufficient to enable most GP registrars to emerge at the end of the training period as competent GPs, in terms of basic knowledge and most clinical skills, but not 'fit for purpose'? Was a different emphasis, with supervision and support, required? This might be provided by a programme, the purpose of which was to enable newly qualified GPs to become 'fit for the purpose' (*see* Box opposite) of working in the primary care system of the NHS.

Fitness for purpose: a description

Health professionals become 'fit for purpose' when they are properly confident and competent to carry out what is regarded as appropriate healthcare provision in the modern setting. For a GP this means:
- having appropriate book knowledge and clinical skills
- knowing how to exercise this knowledge and skill
- knowing how to relate to patients
- knowing how to work in a team
- knowing how to provide services for groups of patients
- knowing how to maintain quality of practice
- knowing how to lay the foundations for lifelong learning.

'Fitness for purpose' is a concept which applies equally to individual healthcare professionals (in this case new GPs) and to the healthcare system in which they work. Both the workers and the organisation must be able to deliver a quality service for patients. The NHS itself must be fit for the purpose of helping the development of its workforce. In part it must do this by providing appropriate opportunities for professional development.

As our new generation of young GPs emerge from their vocational training, it is clear that not being 'fit for purpose' is a real problem. Their undergraduate curriculum may not have addressed the factual and life adaptation skills needed to deal with today's healthcare setting and pace of change. Yes, this deficit is being addressed by modernising the medical undergraduate curriculum. But for today's young GPs this change is too late. The new funding arrangements for protected time for learning at last offer a real opportunity to think about ways of helping post-vocationally trained GPs to further develop themselves, so that fitness for purpose is achieved.

How can we, who are responsible for managing and facilitating these new opportunities for young GPs, best go about our task? We could, at one extreme, look to empower new GPs to explore how best to optimise self-directed learning. We could provide a model which is both more thoughtful and more academic (by academic we mean 'more enquiring, more evidence-based'). We might need to be responsible for the supervision of such reflective learning. Special emphasis would need to be devoted to the resolution of the immediate problems of young doctors, which are usually work-based. Such problems often stem from the real and live difficulties of working with patients. At the other end of the scale, we could offer a purely 'service provision model'. This would be an information-giving and training-based model. We could impart information to new GPs about patients' needs without addressing learners' developmental needs.

But our view is that this latter model would fall short in the long term, with its lack of reflective focus. The model of education, which this chapter will go on to describe, should look to balance the academic and service provision components. It will equip new GPs to move to a reflective self-directed learning method and provide the opportunity to gain and consolidate clinical knowledge and skill of value to the care of their patients.

The strategic importance of HPE

In strategic terms, HPE is of importance for both the recruitment and retention of competent GPs in the new NHS. A framework for HPE provision must be designed to withstand at least three clear challenges.

1   Meeting and supporting the educational needs of new GPs (the transition to independent practice).
2   Assisting new GPs in becoming fit for the purpose of working in the NHS.
3   Enhancing the retention of new GPs in the general practice workforce.

New government funding for HPE came onstream on 1 October 2001, to be managed by Directors of Postgraduate General Practice Education (DsPGPE), and deaneries are now developing their support systems to reach the target group of new GPs. This has required an expansion of the deanery educational network by the appointment of programme directors to support HPE programmes and their participants under the leadership of a lead Associate Dean of Postgraduate General Practice Education (ADPGPE).

Operational developments in HPE

From the historical perspective already discussed in this chapter it can be seen how common themes in HPE, emerging from previous studies, could go on to shape the practicalities of a programme. The structure, content and process of such a programme – what will happen, who will do it, how it will be done and what its aim must be – form the basis of the operational development of HPE.

HPE structure

The structure of a programme for HPE is determined by previous experience (Jackson and Reiss 1998) and the following key factors:

- national policy and the COGPED framework setting the standard
- funding limitations and the number of GPs that may be eligible to enter the scheme
- the educational needs of the GPs
- what the patients and primary care teams will tolerate in terms of reduction in service provision levels whilst educational needs are addressed for GPs
- geographical considerations and sensitivities to locality service needs
- commitment to information technology.

One of the first tasks is to identify new GPs and establish a database that can then support HPE delivery. This presents a number of practical problems because of concurrent changes within the NHS, in organisations managing the necessary data:

- the devolvement of health authority functions to primary care trusts (PCTs)
- the evolution of strategic health authorities (SHAs)
- the establishment of supplementary lists to identify non-principal GPs (some of whom will also be new GPs).

At a time of rapidly expanding personal computing access to the internet, the way in which deaneries support individuals needs to reflect modern information technology (IT) practice. The convenience and speed IT offers individuals in such a setting may be crucial to the perception of being attuned to learners' needs. This may challenge the resources of educational bodies to have IT strategy match user expectation.

The HPE team

Part of the HPE structure is the HPE team. Co-ordinating delivery of HPE to new GPs within these challenges will be the responsibility of educationalists, to be called programme directors (PDs). They will be appointed and managed by the deanery. Their personal qualities, aptitudes and skills will be vital for the success of their mission. They need to be good communicators and facilitators, have educational and clinical experience in primary care, and an ability to network. They will need to make a connection between vocational training schemes (VTS) and continuing professional development (CPD) – the arrangements for lifelong learning for established professionals – to ensure the supportive continuum highlighted earlier. They will need support and supervision in discharging their task, and the time to interact with fellow educators with responsibility in this field. This will give them feedback and stimulate reflection on shared experience. Such a process should both help to generate best practice and inform strategic planning at deanery level.

HPE content

When new GPs assess their educational needs, it is interesting to see how consistent the range of subjects raised is (Abouharb unpublished;[1] Baron *et al.* 2001; Joint Centre for Education in Medicine 1998). This reflects the difficulties new GPs face in transition from the closely supported registrar post to fully fledged independent practice, with potential deficits in knowledge, clinical, management and coping skills. It must also be ensured that new GPs deal with issues of health strategy such as the new national standards of service (National Service Frameworks; NSF), and their local equivalents (Health Improvement Programmes; HImP). New GPs also need to be helped to become sensitive to the patient's perspective.

A working compilation of these into a proposed core curriculum for HPE may be seen in the Appendix to this chapter.

Process of HPE delivery

The key to HPE delivery will be each individual's personal development plan (PDP). As part of national policy, it is intended that PDPs should become a prescribed activity, to be linked with practice and wider needs and planning (DoH 1998). Learning needs assessment (Grant 2002) will form the basis of planning for PDPs and will, therefore, be an early stage in the new GP's learning cycle. Individuals will have unique needs and for the process to be truly effective it must be flexible enough to facilitate each individual's educational journey.

Modes of delivery

Although a range of educational vehicles has been suggested as a way of optimising HPE delivery (Joint Centre for Education in Medicine 1998), an overriding issue is to encourage new GPs to move on from the closely supervised model of VTS day release to a reflective, self-directed learning model. This will serve them better in the longer term.

Funding streams, as laid out in the COGPED framework of the national policy, have ensured protected educational time for new GPs undertaking HPE. There will be service provision support for practices to seek locum cover for new GP learners. This is presently set at 20 whole-day equivalents per year.

---

[1] Higher Professional Education for New GPs North Thames East conference feedback on 8/9/2000 and Higher Professional Education Day for New GPs in London Deanery 11/9/2001.

A much smaller component of the funding is directed to supporting educational activity. The challenge here is how best to use these funds. The range of options for the use of these funds is:

- to fully devolve ownership to individuals to direct as they choose
- to target funds at specific activities, for example supporting self-directed learning groups
- to develop some compromise, which would be overseen in partnership by new GPs and their programme directors.

However these funds are used, and whether new GPs learn within supportive groups or in supervised placements, or on their own, the new GP's PDP will act as the key planning and evaluation document for the following year's educational activity. GPs' PDPs should be built on an awareness or assessment of their learning needs. The programme director will need to make personal contact with new GPs and start the process of facilitating this activity.

This model of supervision has at its heart a dynamic learner-centred relationship between programme director and new GPs. The relative numbers of new GP learners and programme directors is such that it will be difficult to have an exclusive one-to-one relationship here, although to some degree the relationship has to be facilitative and supervisory. Perhaps the element of facilitation and supervision will occur most completely through peer groups? This solution does indeed build on others' experience in the post-vocational scheme support setting. In the study by Bregazzi *et al.* (2000), a one-to-one mentoring model for new GPs in their work setting proved problematic at times, whereas peer support and learning groups were more valued by the participating GPs. In summary, therefore, the proposal for HPE is based on the following.

- Educational supervision by a programme director of individual plans – this may not be conducted on a one-to-one basis and may need to be delegated.
- Emphasis on peer and self-directed learning groups as a most appropriate way to facilitate the learning and development process.

Like our colleagues in other deaneries who are planning HPE, we need to understand how to develop the role of these groups and of individual new GPs within them (Rughani *et al.* 2002). The programme director will need to be facilitative in order to stimulate debate and negotiation in the group so that it can arrive at the most supportive arrangement.

With the bones of the model now outlined, it may be valuable to clarify the learning process and the supportive structure. New GPs are under the professional imperative to ensure that they keep up to date with skills and knowledge and become fit for purpose. Educational supervision and facilitation is provided by the programme director. He may pass this duty on to a third party (for example, a consultant where the young GP is sitting in on clinics.) Equally, the third party may be a peer learning group. So, supervision and support may well be shared with the third party in the setting of a new GP's secondment, or with a learning group that incorporates peer support and supervision. This flexibility thus allows the programme director to both ensure that the learner's needs are addressed and that the learning process takes place in the most appropriate setting.

Programme directors need many skills as gate-keepers of the scheme. They need to maintain the quality and credibility of the educational activity, whilst keeping the option of the mode of delivery firmly in the hands of learners.

Although new GPs may have learning needs not presently addressed in CPD provision, encouraging them to take up existing CPD opportunities that are relevant may serve to reduce the sense of isolation otherwise engendered in learning only as an HPE group. CPD will put them in touch with experienced colleagues whose knowledge base would offer a valuable resource, and potential contacts for a future support network.

HPE and a change in culture

Over the past 20 years there has been a dramatic shift in both the expectations of doctors and their patients of how primary care delivery and its associated educational support should function. This generation of new GPs has grown up and entered the profession since the change in GP contractual regulations in 1990. They often accept that change must occur but are less willing to accept how work in general might affect the quality of their personal and family lives. More females are now choosing a career in primary care, and a greater proportion are choosing to work part time (RCGP 1997).

This change in culture may have been accelerated by a combination of increasing stressors and greater choice. The stressors take the form of increasing litigation, reduction in perceived status and ever-increasing workload. The MB BS qualification may now open doors to other careers with equal if not better rates of pay, potentially generating less angst.

HPE is thus entering the fray at a critical time for recruitment and retention. It may offer the shield to protect new GPs from some of the stressors whilst they develop survival skills. It may also act to bolster new GPs' self-worth as they acquire skills that are relevant to their future practice or to their work within the primary care team. HPE must go some way to addressing these issues. The majority of individuals who opt for a career in general practice do so in the few years after they have qualified as a doctor (Bowler and Jackson 2002). It is therefore important that the positive view they take of this option is maintained through the difficult period of transition after VTS.

Support and supervision for the learning and development of new GPs is important: it is a recognition of the value of the individual within the

NHS. It should help to move the GP toward becoming an adult and self-directed learner. It should establish a reflective approach to personal development. To develop individuals in this way has been the secret of many a successful organisation.

It is in the challenge of delivering HPE that one begins to see the effects of the cultural shift in attitudes to the role and lifestyle of modern-day GPs. Resolving the tension between the personal life and demands of work is one part of the formula. But we must ensure that there are appropriate opportunities for self-development and for becoming 'fit for purpose' so that GPs remain committed and enthusiastic about their chosen work. This may be our best chance to redress the cultural shift that has occurred in our profession over the past generation.

References

Baron R, McKinlay D, Martin J, Ward B and Whiteman I (2001) Higher professional education for GPs in the North West of England – feedback from the first three years. *Ed Prim Care.* **12**: 421–9.

Bowler I and Jackson N (2002) Experiences and career intentions of general practice registrars in Thames deaneries. *BMJ.* **324**: 464–5.

Bregazzi R, Harrison J and van Zwanenberg T (2000) Mentoring new GPs: experience from GP Career Start in County Durham. *Educ Gen Pract.* **11**: 58–64.

Department of Health (1998) *A First Class Service: quality in the new NHS.* HMSO, London.

Freeman G (1997) *LATS Second Annual Report 1996–1997.* Imperial College School of Medicine, London.

Grant J (2002) Learning needs assessment: assessing the need. *BMJ.* **324**: 156–9.

Jackson N and Reiss M (1998) *Higher Professional Education for General Practice. Report on current work in the UK based on completed questionnaires from Directors of Postgraduate General Practice.* Committee of General Practice Education Directors (COGPED), London.

Joint Centre for Education in Medicine (1998) *An Evaluation of Educational Needs and Provision for Doctors within Three Years of Completion of Vocational Training for General Practice.* Joint Centre for Education in Medicine, London.

NHS Executive (1998) *London Initiative Zone Educational Incentive (LIZEI) Scheme, Final Report (Recruitment, Retention, Refreshment and Reflection).* NHS Executive, London.

Royal College of General Practitioners (1965) *Report of a Working Party of Special Vocational Training for General Practice.* RCGP, London.

Royal College of General Practitioners (1997) *The Primary Care Workforce. A descriptive analysis.* RCGP, London.

Rughani A, Tomson M, McFarlane A and Lane P (2002) Continuous professional development – help for new GPs. *Update.* **May**: 742–5.

Appendix 1

Proposed core curriculum for HPE

Performance

- Appraisal and personal development planning
- Preparing for revalidation
- Practice PDPs
- Clinical governance/HImP/NSF

Skills

- IT/presentation skills
- Consultation skills/communication skills/creative problem-solving
- Negotiation skills and assertiveness training/time and stress management
- Audit and research
- Report writing
- Secondary care provision in primary care
- Information-gathering/critical reading skills
- Practising evidence-based medicine

Medicine and the law

- Partnership agreements/joining a practice
- Medico-legal dilemmas
- Ethical dilemmas
- Contractual agreements in the modern NHS (GMS/PMS, etc.)

Practice management and finance

- Practice management/recruitment and employment law
- Personal finance
- Practice finance/accounts and claims

Self-directed personal development/supervision/reflective learning

- Career planning
- Mentoring
- Optimising self-directed learning/self-directed learning groups
- Higher degrees/support for education

CHAPTER 12

Educational supervision in GP vocational training

John Launer

Introduction

The purpose of this chapter is to look at clinical supervision in an educational setting, by looking at vocational training for general practice. I also hope that the chapter may serve to bring a rounded conclusion to the book as a whole, by showing some of the ways that clinical supervision can be established and 'normalised' within primary care. Vocational training is only one example of an area where clinical supervision can be integrated into everyday activities in primary care, in such a way as to alter their style and emphasis quite substantially.

The chapter explores how far the trainer–registrar relationship might involve clinical supervision, exemplified by the different approaches offered in this book. I also want to highlight some of the challenges for clinical supervision in the GP training context, and to suggest ways of addressing these. I write from the perspective of someone who was a GP trainer for many years, and is now involved in teaching established GPs – including trainers – in the skills needed for clinical supervision. By illustrating some of the wider issues that arise in educational supervision, I hope the chapter will also be relevant to training for other primary care professions as well.

Training and supervision

Broadly speaking, the GP vocational training year is the only time in any primary care career when regular, systematic and fairly prolonged case-based discussion is the rule rather than the exception. During the year spent with a GP trainer, most GP registrars get an opportunity at least once a week for some protected time with their trainer, mainly in order to discuss cases that concern them. Many trainers also set aside times for looking at whole surgeries or analysing random cases. In addition, trainers are required to sit in regularly with their registrars and also to review video recordings of consultations; this effectively provides hands-on, intensive discussion of cases of a kind that is almost unknown at any other time during medical training, or indeed in the training of most other medical specialities or primary care disciplines. Beyond the one-to-one engagement with a trainer, the weekly meetings of the local vocational training scheme (possibly with extra 'awaydays' and other similar events) usually offer GP registrars some opportunities for group discussion of cases as well. This may especially have an effect on those who attend an organised three-year VTS rotation. Taken altogether, vocational training therefore potentially provides a richness of opportunities for the kind of practical learning characterised by Donald Schon as involving a reflexive loop between knowledge and experience (Schon 1983).

Given the actual prominence of case discussion in GP vocational training, two things are quite surprising. One is that the term 'clinical supervision' is rarely used in connection with the trainer's role. Indeed, supervision is not usually described as being the core aspect of that role – in very marked contrast to the way that training is understood in professions such as clinical psychology. The other surprising thing is that, although frameworks have been suggested for the trainer–registrar tutorial (Caird and Ogden 2001; Gray 2001) many GP trainers are given little or no explicit instruction in the principles and methods of one-to-one or group supervision. In fact, most of us have embarked on this role simply on the time-honoured basis of 'flying by the seat of our pants'. In practice, this may have involved mimicry of our own trainers or approaches we might have gleaned from a variety of unrelated settings. This unsystematic and unstructured style of supervision also stands in marked contrast to the tradition of formal training for the role of clinical supervisor, as established in some of the other health and welfare professions.

The complexity of the trainer's role

There is one obvious reason why GP trainers are not primarily regarded as clinical supervisors, or formally trained as such. Trainers have many other roles as well. They are educationalists who have to impart a great deal of factual, practical and attitudinal knowledge to their registrars. They are assessors who have to judge their registrars against national standards, and who play a crucial part in accrediting them for entry into the profession. They are clinicians who hold medico-legal responsibility for the acts and omissions of their registrars, and may face disciplinary or service hearings on their registrars' behalf. As employers, they may be accountable to their own partnerships, practice teams and patients for their registrars' performance. Lastly, they are mentors who take on a counselling or even a quasi-parental role in relation to their registrars' career aspirations, and frequently in relation to some aspects of their registrars' personal lives as well. It is, in sum, a complex and challenging relationship in which clinical supervision only plays one part.

In reality, many relationships between GP trainers and their registrars are fairly unproblematic. The registrars are motivated and are well-matched with their trainers, so that successful accreditation may be pretty much a foregone conclusion. In such cases, issues of clinical standards or suitability for employment do not arise. The two parties may be able to treat each other very much as equals and, indeed, trainers may learn as much from their registrars (particularly in the area of recent medical advances) as vice versa. The focus of the relationship may be very much on the kinds of interchange that could be quite accurately defined as clinical supervision. These interchanges might resemble in many ways the various kinds of approach to supervision described elsewhere in this book.

However, most experienced trainers will have at least one registrar at some time in their careers where things are not quite this simple. For example, they may have real doubts about whether a registrar will make the grade clinically, has the right personal attributes for general practice, can adapt to criticism or is capable of learning how to function in a team. In these situations, the role of clinical supervisor becomes more complicated. Case discussions, whether in one-to-one tutorials or group seminars, are influenced by all sorts of anxieties on both sides: anxieties about rejection and failure on the part of the registrar; and anxieties about conflict and exposure to risk on behalf of the trainer. In these situations, it may be necessary to think of the trainer's role in terms of 'modified clinical supervision'; in other words, a role where clinical supervision is significantly mixed with other aspects, such as educational or even disciplinary ones. Even where training is straightforward, there may be discrete moments that are not. There may be times with even the most outstanding registrar when a trainer has to remember who is legally responsible for patients, and has to recall that it is sometimes wise to put experience before enthusiasm.

The sections that follow address a number of different contexts that affect vocational training, concentrating particularly on the year that registrars spend in a GP practice. In looking at these various aspects of training, I try to consider how they may influence the task of clinical supervision or be successfully integrated with it. Each section is illustrated by a fictive 'vignette' loosely based on a number of true problems.

The educational context

Many registrars – although not all – arrive with an adequate level of hospital-based medical knowledge. However, general practice obviously requires much broader knowledge. This includes the vast catalogue of minor but troublesome ailments that are almost never seen in hospital, and it also embraces the natural history of chronic diseases that appear wholly different from their more acute manifestations. These purely medical matters are, of course, only a small proportion of the learning that has to be done. Registrars need to re-orient themselves from a biological to a biographical perspective, and from a timescale of hours or days to one of years or generations – whilst managing individual encounters that are impossibly short. They may need to shed a defensive addiction to diagnostic certainty and to develop instead some other attributes, such as curiosity, puzzlement, patience, improvisation and intuition. Most trainers find that they have to tackle each of these areas of learning to some extent with almost every registrar.

Given the enormity of this list, most trainers will be aware of the tension that arises between the wish to try and impart their knowledge and experience directly, and the need to try and 'bring it forth' through more egalitarian and reflective supervision processes of the kind described elsewhere in this book. One the one hand, there is pressure all the time to revert to an authoritative style of talk – a style dictated not just by the scale of the task but also by much of medical culture, and possibly by the very nature of medical knowledge. There are, self-evidently, medical facts that can only be conveyed didactically: for example, 'This is early chickenpox.' And yet, on the other hand, the most complex and possibly the most important aspects of professional performance may probably be learnt only by finding one's own working style, even if this involves the risk of error. Thus, the pressing reality of the medical setting often means that conversations between trainers and registrars do move from moment to moment between narrative ('What questions had you thought of asking Mr J about his family?') and facts ('If you change him on to amitriptyline, you need to start at a fairly low dose').

Recognising this constant and inevitable tension, what are the ways in which a GP trainer can hold on to a more reflective stance? In other words, how can GP training be sustained as a recognisable form of clinical supervision – of the type promoted in this book – in spite of the imperative to teach a huge professional knowledge base too?

One helpful principle may be to think of the overall context of the training relationship in terms of clinical supervision, but with a recognition that there is often a need to integrate 'moments' of more conventional directive training into this context. The 'moments' may of course be quite long ones, for example if a case discussion exposes an area of considerable ignorance about diagnostic signs or therapeutics. However, thinking of these training moments as digressions, however essential, rather than the core activity of tutorials can help to preserve the ethos as one of 'bringing forth' rather than one of advice-giving.

Going beyond this, it may also be helpful to flag up such 'moments' explicitly when they happen, thus signalling a commitment to the primary aim of the tutorial, namely to help the registrar develop competence and autonomy in all the aspects of the work, not just the informational one. One way this can be done is by naming the temporary shift of context, for example: *'Let's break off for a few minutes to talk about the different antidepressants, but I want to come back afterwards to asking you what you've found out about his home life and his work.'*

Case A

Dr K and her registrar, Dr W, were discussing a complicated case involving an elderly woman with chronic emphysema living in sheltered housing. Their discussion ranged over many topics, but the main ones were (a) any treatment options that might improve the patient's breathing and (b) if it was feasible for the patient to remain in her current flat. In the course of the discussion, Dr K found that there were quite a few gaps in Dr W's knowledge. Dr W did not know about the possibility of domiciliary oxygen or the differences between various kinds of accommodation for the elderly, or the need for consent before referring the patient to the social services department, or the possibility of requesting a visit from the local consultant geriatrician. At a number of points in the discussion, Dr K had to intervene to explain about these things.

At the same time, Dr K tried to hold the discussion within an overall framework of an inquiry into what Dr W understood about the patient's own view of her problems, and what might be done in order to establish what the patient's needs and wishes were. Dr K made sure enough time was left at the end of the tutorial to help Dr W to explore how he might want to proceed in relation to the case, in the light of the knowledge learnt through the discussion.

The assessment context

When vocational training for general practice was originally introduced in the 1960s, it was voluntary. Once it became compulsory under the 1979 regulations its primary purpose changed. It became a formal preparation for professional fitness to practise. As a result of social and political changes since then, assessment has come to have a very high profile in that preparation. In particular, the apparatus of formative and summative assessment has had an effect on both the structure and the experience of GP vocational training. In some circumstances, assessment now dominates trainers' views of their task, and registrars' recollections of their training.

Assessment and clinical supervision are not inherently incompatible. There are many professional trainings where they have to be mixed. Indeed, clinical supervision may be more common in educational settings – and therefore ones where assessment takes place – than in any other. However, there are obvious conflicts between the two activities. Trainees may feel that their performance is covertly being judged under the guise of supervision, or that their qualifications and careers may depend on what they say in apparently 'innocent' case discussions. Conversely, it is hard for educators, however scrupulous, to stop themselves from being influenced by how trainees present themselves in the course of day-to-day exchanges about case work.

What can trainers do in order to prevent the task of assessment contaminating or even overwhelming the opportunities for helpful professional supervision? As discussed above in the educational context, what may be most useful here is an explicit awareness of the two different contexts, and a willingness to address this difference transparently. It may be necessary to specify what is going on at any particular moment; namely, is it really supervision or is it a test? There is nothing wrong with tests, but they need to be labelled as such. When genuine and serious concerns arise about a registrar's competence, it is probably both fairer and more effective to say so openly and at once (as any course organiser and postgraduate dean would advise) than to disguise it as a mock supervision on a case. In practice, this may mean that trainer and registrar have to drop all semblance of clinical supervision from tutorials for a while and replace this by direct instruction and explicit assessment. This also opens the possibility of returning to a more reflective mode of case discussion later, as a marker of success once worries about competence have been allayed.

In most cases, of course, trainers' anxiety about their registrars' competence will be far less, so that the digressions from a reflective kind of interaction are more educational than disciplinary. It is often possible to have fruitful and intelligent discussions about the conflict between assessment and supervision, and how these might be overcome so that the registrar's needs are met and the VTS practice year becomes more of a creative period of personal and professional development rather than a joint exercise in ticking boxes.

To take this a step further, it can be interesting to invite registrars to consider how they might speak or act differently in relation to their trainers, their practices or their work, if assessment were not such a conspicuous dimension of vocational training. This also allows registrars to consider how differently they might wish to behave once they have gained more independence, perhaps as GP principals. It also opens up the important theme of how all medical activity, at whatever level, is to some extent influenced and constrained by assessment contexts of various kinds, even if these arise from professional or legal codes rather than training.

Case B

Dr S was much sought after as a GP trainer for many years. With a local reputation as an unusual and irreverent trainer, he always had his pick of highly competent registrars. In the last few years, however, the number of new VTS entrants in this area has fallen off, and last year Dr S was asked to take on a 'hard to place' registrar from the regional pool.

From the outset, Dr S realised that the registrar, Dr M, was not someone who would have been successful in his VTS application in previous years. His thinking appeared very 'hospitaloid', and he seemed unused to receiving, or digesting, criticism. In spite of some gentle teasing in the first few weeks, he continued to carry out multiple investigations and to make unnecessary referrals without first consulting his trainer. He also persistently, and rather irritably, argued in defence of what he had done on each occasion rather than seeming to be prepared to consider a different way of working.

After a telephone conversation with one of the regional associate deans, Dr S decided to come clean with his registrar by saying that he was unsure whether general practice was the right career for him. He told Dr M explicitly that he would need to make major changes in his performance to persuade him that he could sign his accreditation papers in good faith. He set some clear guidelines, requiring Dr M to confer with him first before ordering X-rays or blood tests, or offering a referral. He also asked Dr M to write down at least three 'hypotheses' after each consultation in order to challenge his apparent certainty.

At first, Dr M responded badly to this confrontation, and seemed to regard it as a professional humiliation. However, over many months, and with several 'near misses' when Dr S thought of asking him to seek another trainer, there was suddenly a conspicuous change in Dr M's performance. For the last two months of the VTS year, Dr S finally felt able to relate to his registrar as a peer, and he was also able to start demonstrating in his tutorials the kind of sceptical, challenging, quirky and ironic style of supervision that his previous registrars had so much appreciated.

The medico-legal context

As practising doctors, both trainers and registrars work within several frameworks of legal liability. These include health authority (or PCT) terms of service, the professional code of conduct supervised by the GMC, and the civil and criminal law. There is, however, a significant difference between a registrar's liability and that of a trainer or the trainer's partners. Registrars are liable only for their own failings. By contrast, trainers are responsible for anything done both by themselves and their registrars. In addition, all the partners in a practice can be held responsible for the action of any other doctor – including a registrar – who has seen their registered patients. This means that a registrar can imperil the reputations, careers and pockets of several doctors in one practice, not to mention their mental equilibrium and professional self-esteem.

In the vast majority of cases, these are not issues of pressing relevance. Although GP trainers have faced hearings of almost every kind on account of the actions and omissions of their registrars, these cases are still rare. For most of the time, anxieties about the various levels of medico-legal liability are probably more of a low background hum rather than a persistent roar. At the same time, the medico-legal context is worth bearing in mind for two reasons.

The first is that legal liability sets the trainer–registrar relationship in its true social context. GP registrars are not independent contractors or autonomous professionals. Being clear and explicit about this may be important. For example, the medico-legal context impinges on the clinical supervision in the same way that education and assessment do. Unless both registrar and trainer are entirely certain about where responsibility ends, case discussions may accidentally convey the impression that registrars can be fully autonomous, or that trainers have no self-interest in what happens to their patients. This can give rise to real risks, By contrast, spelling out the contractual reality of the situation means that trainers can define the genuine constraints on their registrars' freedom. In return, registrars may feel reassured to know that their trainer's motivation for offering adequate training and support goes beyond a vocational one, and includes self-interest too.

The second (and perhaps more important) reason for holding the medico-legal context in mind is that it connects vocational training with its wider purposes: providing the public with a medical service that continues to be safe, effective and ethical, and protecting patients against negligence and malpractice. Seeing the various medico-legal structures in this light sets a positive rather than a defensive background for the task of clinical supervision. Rather than being constricted within a grid of 'Don'ts' and 'Mustn'ts', case discussions may then be guided instead by a consideration of what is ethical and right. This emphasis suggests that the best way that practitioners can protect themselves is by protecting their patients.

Case C
Dr W, a registrar, was on call one morning when he received a request for a home visit to a middle-aged man who had had low back pain for 24 hours. He spoke to the patient's wife on the phone and agreed to carry out the visit. When he later told his trainer, the trainer suggested that it would be more usual to carry out a fuller assessment of the patient by phone, with a view to simply offering advice in the first instance unless there were worrying neurological symptoms. Dr W phoned the family

again and this time asked to speak to the patient himself. Having established that the symptoms gave no rise for medical concern, Dr W said that, instead of visiting, he would simply leave a prescription for painkillers at the reception desk for the patient's wife to collect. He gave advice about rest and gentle mobilisation, and suggested that the patient should phone again in three or four days if the pain was not resolving.

That afternoon, Dr W and his trainer were contacted by the primary care trust who had received a phone complaint from the family that 'the doctor had offered a visit and then changed his mind because he was too busy'. Dr W's trainer responded by saying that he and his registrar would carry out a joint visit immediately. In the course of the visit, the trainer apologised to the family for the apparent withdrawal of an offer to visit. He explained how the second phone call had arisen, and the educational purpose of his original advice to Dr W. Having examined the patient fully (and given the same advice and treatment as before) he said he would take full responsibility for their dissatisfaction and would want any complaint to be made against him and not his registrar.

In a subsequent tutorial, the trainer and registrar spent half an hour reviewing the event reflectively from various angles, including ways of avoiding unnecessary visits without alienating patients, and the risks of withdrawing a prior offer to visit.

The employment context

As organisations, general practices are a peculiar mixture of public service and private business. They are both complex and intimate systems. Registrars who come into practice from hospital jobs, as most do, may suffer something of a culture shock on finding themselves to be both direct employees of their trainers or training practices and members of a small multidisciplinary team. They may know little or nothing about the true role of some of their future colleagues, such as health visitors or community mental health nurses. They may also be unused to relating on a day-to-day basis with a closely knit group of receptionists and secretaries, who are paid far less than they are but may be of a similar age to their own parents. They are likely to be ignorant of whole areas of relevant knowledge, such as employment law, health and safety at work or accounts. A great deal of the educational content of the vocational training year is therefore usually related to the nature of the practice as an organisation, and the regulations and conventions by which it functions.

Because of this, clinical supervision in tutorials and day-to-day conversations may need to focus as much on 'cases' involving teamwork or staff relationships as on patients. Often, the successful management of cases depends on the successful management of the working network as well, so that supervision has to encompass both at the same time. In much clinical supervision, discussion will weave in and out of matters directly related to the patient, and matters arising from the way that the local health service network (both within and around the practice) operates (Launer 2002).

When employment problems do arise with trainees, such as lateness, disrespect to clerical staff or conflict with other professionals, clarity and explicitness about the organisational context may once again make a difference. Problems like these are not just educational and assessment issues. Even in the absence of any vocational training context, an employee might expect to be called to account for them. In order to free up the trainer–registrar relationship for its more important purposes, therefore, it can sometimes be helpful to define employment as the main context in which these and similar problems will be addressed. Again, a clearly stated distinction between a discussion of employment difficulties and a conversation that is firmly identified as clinical supervision can help trainers to avoid blurring the two.

Case D

For personal and family reasons, Dr F decided to enter general practice in middle age after ten years as a consultant gynaecologist in another part of the country. Because of her previous experience in surgery, paediatrics, and accident and emergency, she was exempted from any further hospital training but still needed to complete a year in a general practice. At first her training went extremely well, and the practice appreciated her maturity and took advantage of her specialist knowledge. However, after a few weeks several members of the office staff disclosed to the practice manager that she was treating them in quite a dictatorial manner. The manager also discovered that, although Dr F seemed to be making herself very popular with the doctors, she was alienating the non-medical members of the team by persistent brusqueness, which in some cases they experienced as harassment.

Her trainer, Dr R, talked to his colleagues about how to deal with this problem, and in particular whether it should be seen as a purely educational matter or whether it was taking on the dimensions of a significant employment problem. They decided it should be handled on both levels. Dr R first alerted his registrar to the complaints about her manner. He explained to her that the practice manager held a responsibility to ensure that all practice personnel were on reasonable terms, and would now be monitoring any further incidents on behalf of the partnership. He made it clear that this had to be construed as 'a verbal warning' and suggested that Dr F should seek some independent advice to make sure she understood its implications. At the same time, he set aside a great deal of time in tutorials to explore with Dr F the differences in working culture between hospitals and general practices, and the difficulties she might be experiencing in adjusting to a junior position after a decade in authority. The combination of formal caution and personal support seemed to work well, and Dr F ended up feeling she had learnt a lot from having been tackled about a habitual manner she later described as 'a bit like a dinosaur at a dinner party.'

The pastoral context

The trainer–registrar relationship is, above all, a human one. Many such relationships turn into lifelong friendships. Nearly all are characterised by a closeness that goes beyond professional contact and includes meeting and getting to know other family members on both sides. Because most trainers are at an age where they are likely to be settled domestically, and many registrars are not, the period of vocational training may well be one in which the trainer has to display protectiveness and tolerance while the registrar suffers, for example, the vicissitudes of an uncertain romance or the sleeplessness of early parenthood. Of course, sudden personal or family illness, loss or bereavement can occur on either side in a way that can both challenge and deepen the relationship.

Trainers and registrars will vary enormously in how far they wish the contact with their registrars to involve a warm emotional bond or some degree of personal disclosure. There will be an instinctive adjustment to a different level with each successive registrar. One way of framing the process of adjustment, and of learning about each other as human beings, is to understand this in terms of 'modelling' the role of educator, and indeed of doctor. In other words, by their ability both to open up emotionally and to retain appropriate reserve, trainers are demonstrating something about the need for balance in an educational stance, and in the medical stance as well. In the context of clinical supervision, just as in consultations with patients, an important question to guide any impulse to share personal feelings or information is often: 'How will this help with the task in hand?'

It is impossible to offer guidelines to answer that question. Experienced trainers will no doubt be able to recall occasions when they went too far, and declared to their registrars that they held strong prejudices against certain colleagues or patients, for example, when it might have been more helpful (if less spontaneous) to conceal this. By contrast, they may also recall encounters with some registrars that seemed to be impoverished by a shared inability to discuss things except in a rather stilted, over-respectful fashion. Since clinical supervision is of its essence a responsive interchange, evolving through the exploration of ideas and experimentation, mistakes of tone and content are probably both inevitable and productive.

Case E

In the course of his registrar year, Dr O had to travel to and from Ireland a number of times in order to visit his father who had suffered a serious stroke. After some months, his father died and he had to take three weeks off to attend the funeral and care for his bereaved mother. During the whole course of the training, considerable periods of time were taken up in some way or another with the father's illness and death. There were the practical arrangements to consider (including cancelled surgeries and the need to cover the training curriculum adequately) as well as the emotional impact on Dr O of seeing his father severely disabled, and then his mother grieving intensely. During much of this time, his trainer Dr R effectively became a comforter and friend, often inviting his registrar round to his house for a meal. Dr R was himself aware that, by responding at a human level rather than in a detached way, he was acting from a part of his personality and his own experience of bereavement that he often drew on when helping patients deal with extreme circumstances.

During the weeks and months of disruption to the training year, Dr R mentioned on a few occasions that it might be necessary to extend the time that Dr O spent in the practice, in order to satisfy the vocational training requirements. However, he also made it clear that his registrar's personal and family needs should come first, and that he had no doubt that it would be possible to set up the practical and financial arrangements for such an extension. When Dr O eventually returned from his compassionate leave, he was relieved to find that his trainer had already put these arrangements in place.

Conclusion

GP vocational training cannot be thought of simply in terms of clinical supervision. It combines many other elements or contexts. Sometimes these are relatively clear, but sometimes they overlap in any number of ways. No doubt there are many occasions when encounters in vocational training take place in 'grey areas' that cannot in any way be analysed according to the fairly simple schema I have offered above, or addressed by the suggestions I have offered.

Nevertheless, what I have tried to suggest in this chapter, and to demonstrate, is that it may be useful to think of clinical supervision as lying at the core of vocational training, and to see the other aspects of training as modifying it but ideally not displacing it. All the other aspects of the trainer–registrar relationship, such as the ones I have enumerated, have to be taken very seriously. Indeed, clinical supervision may not be possible in vocational training unless these are each named, used and opened up for discussion. However, the advantage of according primacy to clinical supervision as a mode of thinking and of discourse in vocational training, and as a constant day-to-day aspiration, is that it preserves the integrity of the experience in terms of its original purpose: namely, to prepare practitioners for practice. Clinical supervision takes training beyond the point that merely satisfies the requirements of official agencies. Instead, it addresses the lived experience of patients and professionals, in all its indescribable complexity, and thus provides a true apprenticeship.

As I suggested at the beginning of this chapter, it may also be worth thinking of vocational training, and the opportunities it provides for clinical supervision, as a model for thinking about primary care as a whole, across all its different professions and varying activities. There are many other things going on every day in primary care, including team meetings and a whole range of educational activities, that offer occasions for introducing case-based discussions, and promoting them as an effective way of learning for adult professionals. The movement to promote clinical supervision and support throughout primary care may in the end be successful not so much through organisational change but rather as a result of incremental shifts in the way we think about our teaching, our learning and our practice.

References

Caird R and Ogden J (2001) Understanding the tutorial in general practice: towards the development of an assessment tool. *Educ Gen Pract.* 12: 57–61.

Gray R (2001) A framework for looking at the trainer/registrar tutorial in general practice. *Educ Gen Pract.* **12**: 153–62.

Launer J (2002) *Narrative-based Primary Care.* Radcliffe Medical Press, Oxford.

Schon D (1983) *The Reflective Practitioner: how professionals think in action.* Temple Smith, London.

Index